ALSO BY GARY TAUBES

Good Calories, Bad Calories:
Challenging the Conventional Wisdom on Diet,
Weight Control, and Disease

Bad Science:
The Short Life and Weird Times of Cold Fusion

Nobel Dreams:
Power, Deceit and the Ultimate Experiment

WHY WE GET FAT

WHY WE GET
FAT

And What to Do About It

GARY TAUBES

ALFRED A. KNOPF   NEW YORK   2011

THIS IS A BORZOI BOOK
PUBLISHED BY ALFRED A. KNOPF

All rights reserved. Published in the United States by
Alfred A. Knopf, a division of Random House, Inc., New York, and in
Canada by Random House of Canada Limited, Toronto.
www.aaknopf.com

Knopf, Borzoi Books, and the colophon are registered trademarks
of Random House, Inc.

Library of Congress Cataloging-in-Publication Data
Taubes, Gary.
Why we get fat and what to do about it / Gary Taubes.
p. cm.
Includes bibliographical references and index.
ISBN 978-0-307-27270-6
1. Low-carbohydrate diet. 2. Weight loss. 3. Obesity—Etiology. I. Title.
RM237.73.T39 2011
613.7'12—dc22 2010034248

Jacket photograph by Mark Dye.
Jacket design by Barbara de Wilde.

Manufactured in the United States of America
Published January 4, 2011
Second Printing, February 2011

This book is not intended as a substitute for medical advice of physicians.
The information given here is designed to help you make informed decisions
about your health. However, before starting the dietary recommendations in
this book or any other diet regimen, you should consult your physician.

To N.N.T.

CONTENTS

AUTHOR'S NOTE

This book has been in the works for more than a decade. It began with a series of investigative articles that I wrote for the journal *Science* and then the *New York Times Magazine* on the surprisingly dismal state of nutrition and chronic-disease research. It is an extension and distillation of the five years of further research that became my previous book, *Good Calories, Bad Calories* (2007). Its arguments were honed in lectures at medical schools, universities, and research institutions throughout the United States and Canada.

What I tried to make clear in *Good Calories, Bad Calories* was that nutrition and obesity research lost its way after the Second World War with the evaporation of the European community of scientists and physicians that did the pioneering work in those disciplines. It has since resisted all attempts to correct it. As a result, the individuals involved in this research have not only wasted decades of time, effort, and money but have done incalculable damage along the way. Their beliefs have remained impervious to an ever-growing body of evidence that refutes them while being embraced by public-health authorities and translated into precisely the wrong advice about what to eat and, more important, what not to eat if we want to maintain a healthy weight and live a long and healthy life.

I decided to write *Why We Get Fat* largely because of two common responses that I receive to *Good Calories, Bad Calories*.

The first comes from those researchers who made an effort to understand the arguments in *Good Calories, Bad Calories*, who read the book or listened to one of my lectures or discussed these ideas with me directly. I'm often told by these people that what

I'm saying about why we get fat, and about the dietary causes of heart disease, diabetes, and other chronic diseases, makes significant sense. It certainly could be right, they say, with the unspoken implication that what we've been told for the past half-century certainly could be wrong. We all agree that these competing ideas should be tested.

I believe, though, that this is an urgent matter. If so many people are getting fat and diabetic in large part because we've been getting the wrong advice, we should not be dawdling about determining that with certainty. The disease burdens of obesity and diabetes are already overwhelming not only hundreds of millions of individuals but our health-care systems as well.

Even if these researchers do see the need to address the problem immediately, though, they have obligations and legitimate interests elsewhere, including being funded for other research. With luck, the ideas discussed in *Good Calories, Bad Calories* may be rigorously tested in the next twenty years. If confirmed, it will be another decade or so after that, at least, before our public-health authorities actively change their official explanation for why we get fat, how that leads to illness, and what we have to do to avoid or reverse those fates. As I was told by a professor of nutrition at New York University after one of my lectures, the kind of change I'm advocating could take a lifetime to be accepted.

That is simply too long to wait to get the right answers to these critical questions. So this book was written in part to speed up the process. I offer here the arguments against the conventional wisdom distilled down to their essence. If they certainly could be right, then let's test them, and let's do it sooner rather than later.

The other response I get frequently is from those lay readers, as well as an encouraging number of physicians, nutritionists, researchers, and health administrators, who say that they read *Good Calories, Bad Calories* or listened to my lectures, found the logic and the evidence compelling, and embraced the message implicit in it. They tell me their lives and their health have been transformed in ways they didn't think possible. They have lost weight almost effortlessly and have kept it off. Their risk factors for heart disease have improved dramatically. Some say they no longer need their hypertension and diabetes medications. They feel better and have more energy. Put simply, they feel healthy for the first time in far too long. You can see these kinds of comments on the Amazon web page for *Good Calories, Bad Calories*, where they represent a large proportion of the several hundred personal reviews at the site.

These comments, e-mails, and letters have often come with a request. *Good Calories, Bad Calories* is lengthy (nearly five hundred pages), dense with science and historical context, and densely annotated, all of which I believe was necessary to initiate a meaningful dialogue with the experts and assure that they (or any reader) take nothing I say on trust alone. The book demands that the reader devote considerable time and attention to following the evidence and the arguments. For this reason, many who read it have asked me to write another book, one that their husbands or wives, their aging parents, or their friends and siblings can read without difficulty. Many physicians have asked me to write a book that they can give to their patients, or even to their fellow physicians, a book that doesn't require such an investment of time and effort.

So this is the other reason I wrote *Why We Get Fat*. I hope by reading it you will understand, perhaps for the first time, why we do get fat and what to do about it.

My one request is that you think critically while you're reading. I want you to keep asking yourself as you read whether what I'm saying really makes sense. To steal a phrase from Michael Pollan, this book is intended to be a thinker's manifesto. Its goal is to refute some of the misconceptions that pass for public-health and medical advice in this country and around the world, and to arm you with the necessary information and logic to take your health and well-being into your own hands.

One word of caution though: If you accept my arguments as valid and change your diet accordingly, you may be going against

your doctor's advice, and certainly that of the health organizations and government agencies that dictate the consensus opinion
on what constitutes a healthy diet. In that sense, you read this
book and act on it at your own risk. That situation can be recti-
fied, though, by giving this book to your physician when you're
done reading it, so that he or she, too, can decide who and what to
believe. And you might give it to your congressional representatives as well, because the rising tides of obesity and diabetes in the
United States and throughout the world are indeed massive
public-health problems, not just our own individual burdens to
bear. It would help if our elected representatives actually understood how we got into this situation, so they could act finally to
resolve it, rather than perpetuate it.

—G.T., September 2010

WHY WE GET FAT

INTRODUCTION

The Original Sin

In 1934, a young German pediatrician named Hilde Bruch moved to America, settled in New York City, and was "startled," as she later wrote, by the number of fat children she saw—"really fat ones, not only in clinics, but on the streets and subways, and in schools." Indeed, fat children in New York were so conspicuous that other European immigrants would ask Bruch about it, assuming that she would have an answer. What is the matter with American children? they would ask. Why are they so bloated and blown up? Many would say they'd never seen so many children in such a state.

Today we hear such questions all the time, or we ask them ourselves, with the continual reminders that we are in the midst of an epidemic of obesity (as is the entire developed world). Similar questions are asked about fat adults. Why are *they* so bloated and blown up? Or you might ask yourself: Why am I?

But this was New York City in the mid-1930s. This was two decades before the first Kentucky Fried Chicken and McDonald's franchises, when fast food as we know it today was born. This was half a century before supersizing and high-fructose corn syrup. More to the point, 1934 was the depths of the Great Depression, an era of soup kitchens, bread lines, and unprecedented unemployment. One in every four workers in the United States was unemployed. Six out of every ten Americans were living in poverty. In New York City, where Bruch and her fellow immigrants were astonished by the adiposity of the local children,

3

one in four children were said to be malnourished. How could this be?

A year after arriving in New York, Bruch established a clinic at Columbia University's College of Physicians and Surgeons to treat obese children. In 1939, she published the first of a series of reports on her exhaustive studies of the many obese children she had treated, although almost invariably without success. From interviews with her patients and their families, she learned that these obese children did indeed eat excessive amounts of food— no matter how much either they or their parents might initially deny it. Telling them to eat less, though, just didn't work, and no amount of instruction or compassion, counseling, or exhortations—of either children or parents—seemed to help.

It was hard to avoid, Bruch said, the simple fact that these children had, after all, spent their entire lives trying to eat in moderation and so control their weight, or at least thinking about eating less than they did, and yet they remained obese. Some of these children, Bruch reported, "made strenuous efforts to lose weight, practically giving up on living to achieve it." But maintaining a lower weight involved "living on a continuous semi-starvation diet," and they just couldn't do it, even though obesity made them miserable and social outcasts.

One of Bruch's patients was a fine-boned girl in her teens, "literally disappearing in mountains of fat." This young girl had spent her life fighting both her weight and her parents' attempts to help her slim down. She knew what she had to do, or so she believed, as did her parents—she had to eat less—and the struggle to do this defined her existence. "I always knew that life depended on your figure," she told Bruch. "I was always unhappy and depressed when gaining [weight]. There was nothing to live for. . . . I actually hated myself. I just could not stand it. I didn't want to look at myself. I hated mirrors. They showed how fat I was. . . . It never made me feel happy to eat and get fat—but I never could see a solution for it and so I kept on getting fatter."

. . .

Like Bruch's fine-boned girl, those of us who are overweight or obese will spend much of our lives trying to eat less, or at least eat not too much. Sometimes we succeed, sometimes we fail, but the fight goes on. For some, like Bruch's patients, the battle begins in childhood. For others, it starts in college with the freshman twenty, that cushion of fat that appears around waist and hips while spending the first year away from home. Still others begin to realize in their thirties or forties that being lean is no longer the effortless achievement it once was.

Should we be fatter than the medical authorities would prefer, and should we visit a doctor for any reason, that doctor is likely to suggest more or less forcefully that we do something about it. Obesity and overweight, so we'll be told, are associated with an increased risk of virtually every chronic disease that ails us—heart disease, stroke, diabetes, cancer, dementia, asthma. We'll be instructed to exercise regularly, to diet, to eat less, as though the thought of doing so, the desire to do so, would never otherwise have crossed our minds. "More than in any other illness," as Bruch said about obesity, "the physician is called upon only to do a special trick, to make the patient do something—stop eating—after it has already been proved that he cannot do it."

The physicians of Bruch's era weren't thoughtless, and the doctors of today are not, either. They merely have a flawed belief system—a paradigm—that stipulates that the reason we get fat is clear and incontrovertible, as is the cure. We get fat, our physicians tell us, because we eat too much and/or move too little, and so the cure is to do the opposite. If nothing else, we should eat "not too much," as Michael Pollan famously prescribes in his best-selling book *In Defense of Food*, and this will suffice. At least we won't get fatter still. This is what Bruch described in 1957 as the "prevalent American attitude that the problem [of obesity] is simply one of eating more than the body needs," and now it's the prevalent attitude worldwide.

We can call this the "calories-in/calories-out" or the "overeating" paradigm of excess fat—the "energy balance" paradigm, if we want to get technical. "The fundamental cause of obesity and overweight," as the World Health Organization says, "is an energy imbalance between calories consumed on one hand, and calories expended on the other hand."* We get fat when we take in more energy than we expend (a positive energy balance, in the scientific terminology), and we get lean when we expend more than we take in (a negative energy balance). Food is energy, and we measure that energy in the form of calories. So, if we take in more calories than we expend, we get fatter. If we take in fewer calories, we get leaner.

This way of thinking about our weight is so compelling and so pervasive that it is virtually impossible nowadays *not* to believe it. Even if we have plenty of evidence to the contrary—no matter how much of our lives we've spent consciously trying to eat less and exercise more without success—it's more likely that we'll question our own judgment and our own willpower than we will this notion that our adiposity is determined by how many calories we consume and expend.

My favorite example of this thinking came from a well-respected exercise physiologist, a co-author of a set of physical-

---

*Such official pronouncements are effectively universal. Here are a few more: The U.S. Centers for Disease Control: "Weight management is all about balance—balancing the number of calories you consume with the number of calories your body uses or 'burns off.'" The U.K. Medical Research Council: "Although the rise in obesity cannot be attributed to any single factor, it is the simple imbalance between energy in (through the food choices we make) and energy out (mainly through physical activity) which is the cause." INSERM, the French National Institute of Health and Medical Research: "Excess body weight and obesity always result from an imbalance between energy intake and energy expenditure." The German Federal Ministry of Health: "Overweight is the result of too much energy consumed compared with the energy expended."

activity and health guidelines that were published in August 2007 by the American Heart Association and the American College of Sports Medicine. This fellow told me that he personally had been "short, fat, and bald" when he first took up distance running in the 1970s, and now he was in his late sixties and was "short, *fatter*, and bald." In the intervening years, he said, he had gained thirty-odd pounds and run maybe eighty thousand miles—the equivalent, more or less, of running three times around the Earth (at the equator). He believed that there was a limit to how much exercise could help him maintain his weight, but he also believed he would be fatter still if he hadn't been running.

When I asked him whether he really thought he might be leaner had he run even more, maybe run four times around the planet instead of three, he said, "I don't see how I could have been more active. I had no time to do more. But if I could have gone out over the last couple of decades for two to three hours a day, maybe I would not have gained this weight." And the point is that maybe he would have anyway, but he just couldn't wrap his head around that possibility. As sociologists of science would say, he was trapped in a paradigm.

Over the years, this calories-in/calories-out paradigm of excess fat has proved to be remarkably resistant to any evidence to the contrary. Imagine a murder trial in which one credible witness after another takes the stand and testifies that the suspect was elsewhere at the time of the killing and so had an airtight alibi, and yet the jurors keep insisting that the defendant is guilty, because that's what they believed when the trial began.

Consider the obesity epidemic. Here we are as a population getting fatter and fatter. Fifty years ago, one in every eight or nine Americans would have been officially considered obese, and today it's one in every three. Two in three are now considered overweight, which means they're carrying around more weight than the public-health authorities deem to be healthy. Children are fatter, adolescents are fatter, even newborn babies are emerging from the womb fatter. Throughout the decades of this obesity epidemic, the calories-in/calories-out, energy-balance notion has held sway, and so the health officials assume that either we're not paying attention to what they've been telling us—eat less and exercise more—or we just can't help ourselves.

Malcolm Gladwell discussed this paradox in *The New Yorker* in 1998. "We have been told that we must not take in more calories than we burn, that we cannot lose weight if we don't exercise consistently," he wrote. "That few of us are able to actually follow this advice is either our fault or the fault of the advice. Medical orthodoxy, naturally, tends toward the former position. Diet books tend toward the latter. Given how often the medical orthodoxy has been wrong in the past, that position is not, on its face, irrational. It's worth finding out whether it is true."

After interviewing the requisite number of authorities, Gladwell decided that it was our fault, that we simply "lack the discipline . . . or the wherewithal" to eat less and move more—although for some of us, he suggested, bad genes extract a greater price in adiposity for our moral failings.

I will argue in this book that the fault lies entirely with the medical orthodoxy—both the belief that excess fat is caused by consuming excess calories, and the advice that stems from it. I'm going to argue that this calories-in/calories-out paradigm of adiposity is nonsensical: that we don't get fat because we eat too much and move too little, and that we can't solve the problem or prevent it by consciously doing the opposite. This is the original sin, so to speak, and we're never going to solve our own weight problems, let alone the societal problems of obesity and diabetes and the diseases that accompany them, until we understand this and correct it.

I don't mean to imply, though, that there is a magic recipe to losing weight, or at least not one that doesn't include sacrifice. The question is, what has to be sacrificed?

The first part of this book will present the evidence against the calories-in/calories-out hypothesis. It will discuss many of the observations, the facts of life, that this concept fails to explain, why we came to believe it anyway, and what mistakes were made as a result.

The second part of this book will present the way of thinking about obesity and excess fat that European medical researchers came to accept just prior to the Second World War. They argued, as I will, that it is absurd to think about obesity as *caused* by overeating, because anything that makes people grow—whether in height or in weight, in muscle or in fat—will make them overeat. Children, for example, don't grow taller because they eat voraciously and consume more calories than they expend. They eat so much—overeat—because they're growing. They *need* to take in more calories than they expend. The reason children grow is that they're secreting hormones that make them do so—in this case, growth hormone. And there is every reason to believe that the growth of our fat tissue leading to overweight and obesity is also driven and controlled by hormones.

So, rather than define obesity as a disorder of energy balance or eating too much, as the experts have for the past half-century, these European medical researchers started from the idea that obesity is fundamentally a disorder of excess fat accumulation. This is what a philosopher would call "first principles." It's so obviously true that it seems almost meaningless to say it. But once we do, then the natural question to ask is, what regulates fat accumulation? Because whatever hormones or enzymes work to increase our fat accumulation naturally—just as growth hormone makes children grow—are going to be the very likely suspects on which to focus to determine why some of us get fat and others don't.

Regrettably, the European medical-research community barely survived the Second World War, and these physicians and their ideas about obesity weren't around in the late 1950s and early 1960s, when this question of what regulates fat accumulation was answered. As it turns out, two factors will essentially determine how much fat we accumulate, both having to do with the hormone insulin.

First, when insulin levels are elevated, we accumulate fat in our fat tissue; when these levels fall, we liberate fat from the fat tissue and burn it for fuel. This has been known since the early 1960s and has never been controversial. Second, our insulin levels are effectively determined by the carbohydrates we eat—not entirely, but for all intents and purposes. The more carbohydrates we eat, and the easier they are to digest and the sweeter they are, the more insulin we will ultimately secrete, meaning that the level of it in our bloodstream is greater and so is the fat we retain in our fat cells. "Carbohydrate is driving insulin is driving fat," is how George Cahill, a former professor of medicine at Harvard Medical School, recently described this to me. Cahill had done some of the early research on the regulation of fat accumulation in the 1950s, and then he coedited an eight-hundred-page American Physiological Society compendium of this research that was published in 1965.

In other words, the science itself makes clear that hormones, enzymes, and growth factors regulate our fat tissue, just as they do everything else in the human body, and that we do not get fat because we overeat; we get fat because the carbohydrates in our diet make us fat. The science tells us that obesity is ultimately the result of a hormonal imbalance, not a caloric one—specifically, the stimulation of insulin secretion caused by eating easily digestible, carbohydrate-rich foods: refined carbohydrates, including flour and cereal grains, starchy vegetables such as potatoes, and sugars, like sucrose (table sugar) and high-fructose corn syrup. These carbohydrates literally make us fat, and by driving us to accumulate fat, they make us hungrier and they make us sedentary.

This is the fundamental reality of why we fatten, and if we're to get lean and stay lean we'll have to understand and accept it, and, perhaps more important, our doctors are going to have to understand and acknowledge it, too.

If your goal in reading this book is simply to be told the answer to the question "What do I do to remain lean or lose the excess fat

I have?" then this is it: stay away from carbohydrate-rich foods, and the sweeter the food or the easier it is to consume and digest—liquid carbohydrates like beer, fruit juices, and sodas are probably the worst—the more likely it is to make you fat and the more you should avoid it.

This is certainly not a new message. Until the 1960s, as I'll discuss later, it was the conventional wisdom. Carbohydrate-rich foods—bread, pasta, potatoes, sweets, beer—were seen to be uniquely fattening, and if you wanted to avoid being fat, you didn't eat them. Since then, it has been the message of an unending string of often best-selling diet books. But this essential fact has been so abused, and the relevant science so distorted or misinterpreted, both by proponents of these "carbohydrate-restricted" diets and by those who insist that they are dangerous fads (the American Heart Association among them) that I want to lay it out once more. If you find the argument sufficiently compelling that you want to change your diet accordingly, then all the better. I will give some advice on how to do so, based on the lessons learned by clinicians who have years of experience using these diets to treat their overweight and often diabetic patients.

In the more than six decades since the end of the Second World War, when this question of what causes us to fatten—calories or carbohydrates—has been argued, it has often seemed like a religious issue rather than a scientific one. So many different belief systems enter into the question of what constitutes a healthy diet that the scientific question—why do we get fat?—has gotten lost along the way. It's been overshadowed by ethical, moral, and sociological considerations that are valid in themselves and certainly worth discussing but have nothing to do with the *science* itself and arguably no place in a scientific inquiry.

Carbohydrate-restricted diets typically (if not, perhaps, ideally) replace the carbohydrates in the diet with large or at least larger portions of animal products—beginning with eggs for breakfast and moving to meat, fish, or fowl for lunch and dinner. The implications of that are proper to debate. Isn't our dependence on animal products already bad for the environment, and won't it just get worse? Isn't livestock production a major contributor to global warming, water shortages, and pollution? When thinking about a healthy diet, shouldn't we think about what's good for the planet as well as what's good for us? Do we have a right to kill animals for our food or put them to work for us in producing it? Isn't the only morally and ethically defensible lifestyle a vegetarian one or even a vegan one?

These are all important questions that need to be addressed, as individuals and as a society. But they have no place in the scientific and medical discussion of why we get fat. And that's what I am setting out to explore here—just as Hilde Bruch did more than seventy years ago. Why are we fat? Why are our children fat? What can we do about it?

BOOK I

Biology, Not Physics

1

Why Were They Fat?

Imagine you're serving on a jury. The defendant is accused of some heinous crime. The prosecuting attorney has evidence that he says implicates the defendant beyond reasonable doubt. He says the evidence is as clear as day and that you must vote to convict. This criminal must be put beyond bars, you're told, because he's a threat to society.

The defense attorney is arguing just as vehemently that the evidence is not so clear-cut. The defendant has an alibi, albeit not one that's airtight. There are fingerprints at the crime scene that don't match the defendant's. He suggests the police may have mishandled the forensic evidence (the DNA and hair samples). The defense argues that the case is not nearly as definitive as the prosecutor has led you to believe. If you have reasonable doubt, as you should, you must acquit, he says. If you put an innocent man behind bars, you're told, not only do you do that person an incalculable injustice, but you leave the guilty party free to strike again.

In the jury room, your job is to assess the claims and counterclaims and make a decision based solely on the evidence. It doesn't matter what your inclinations might have been when the trial began. It doesn't matter whether you thought the defendant looked guilty or didn't appear to be the kind of person who could commit such a horrible act. All that matters is the evidence and whether or not it's convincing.

One thing we know about criminal justice is that innocent people are often convicted of crimes they didn't commit, despite a judiciary system that is dedicated to avoiding just that outcome. A common theme in the litany of justice poorly served is that those wrongly convicted are typically the obvious suspects. Their conviction feels right; evidence that might exculpate them is more easily disregarded. Complicated questions are pushed aside, as is evidence that just might free them after their conviction.

It would be nice to think that science and scientists don't make such errors, but they happen all the time. It's human nature. The methods of science are supposed to guard against the adoption of false convictions, but these methods aren't always followed, and even when they are, inferring the truth about nature and the universe is a difficult business. Common sense can be an effective guide, but as Voltaire pointed out in his *Dictionnaire philosophique*, common sense isn't all that common, even among scientists, and often what science tells us is that the things that appear to be common sense aren't. The sun does not revolve around the earth, for example, despite superficial appearances to the contrary.

What sets science and the law apart from religion is that nothing is expected to be taken on faith. We're encouraged to ask whether the evidence actually supports what we're being told to believe—or what we grew up believing—and we're allowed to ask whether we're hearing all the evidence or just some small prejudicial part of it. If our beliefs aren't supported by the evidence, then we're encouraged to alter our beliefs.

It is surprisingly easy to find evidence that refutes the conviction that we get fat because we take in more calories than we expend—that is, because we overeat. In most of science, skeptical appraisals of the evidence are considered a fundamental requirement to make progress. In nutrition and public health, however, they are seen by many as counterproductive, because they undermine efforts to promote behaviors that the authorities believe, rightly or wrongly, are good for us.

But our health (and our weight) are at stake here, so let's take a look at this evidence and see where it leads us. Imagine we're on a jury charged with deciding whether or not it's overeating—taking in more calories than we expend—that is responsible for the "crime" of obesity and overweight.

A convenient starting point is the obesity epidemic. Ever since researchers at the Centers for Disease Control and Prevention (CDC) broke the news in the mid-1990s that the epidemic was upon us, authorities have blamed it on overeating and sedentary behavior and blamed those two factors on the relative wealth of modern societies.

"Improved prosperity" caused the epidemic, aided and abetted by the food and entertainment industries, as the New York University nutritionist Marion Nestle explained in the journal *Science* in 2003. "They turn people with expendable income into consumers of aggressively marketed foods that are high in energy but low in nutritional value, and of cars, television sets, and computers that promote sedentary behavior. Gaining weight is good for business."

The Yale University psychologist Kelly Brownell coined the term "toxic environment" to describe the same notion. Just as the residents of Love Canal or Chernobyl lived in toxic environments that encouraged cancer growth (chemicals in the groundwater and radioactivity), the rest of us, Brownell says, live in a toxic environment "that encourages overeating and physical inactivity." Obesity is the natural consequence. "Cheeseburgers and French fries, drive-in windows and supersizes, soft drinks and candy, potato chips and cheese curls, once unusual, are as much our background as trees, grass, and clouds," he says. "Few children walk or bike to school; there is little physical education; computers, video games, and televisions keep children inside and inactive; and parents are reluctant to let children roam free to play."

In other words, we are told, too much money, too much food, too easily available, plus too many incentives to be sedentary—or too little need to be physically active—have caused the obesity epidemic. The World Health Organization uses the identical logic to explain the obesity epidemic worldwide, blaming it on rising incomes, urbanization, "shifts toward less physically demanding work... moves toward less physical activity... and more passive leisure pursuits." Obesity researchers now use a quasi-scientific term to describe exactly this condition: they refer to the "obesigenic" environment in which we now live, meaning an environment that is prone to turning lean people into fat ones.

One piece of evidence that needs to be considered in this context, however, is the well-documented fact that being fat is associated with poverty, not prosperity—certainly in women, and often in men. The poorer we are, the fatter we're likely to be. This was first reported in a survey of New Yorkers—midtown Manhattanites—in the early 1960s: obese women were six times more likely to be poor than rich; obese men, twice as likely. It's been confirmed in virtually every study since, both in adults and in children, including those same CDC surveys that revealed the existence of the obesity epidemic.*

Can it be possible that the obesity epidemic is caused by prosperity, so the richer we get, the fatter we get, and that obesity associates with poverty, so the poorer we are, the more likely we are to be fat? It's not impossible. Maybe poor people don't have the peer pressure that rich people do to remain thin. Believe it or not, this has been one of the accepted explanations for this apparent paradox. Another commonly accepted explanation for the association between obesity and poverty is that fatter women marry down in social class and so collect at the bottom rungs of the ladder; thinner women marry up. A third is that poor people don't have the

---

*In 1968, George McGovern, a U.S. senator, chaired a series of congressional hearings in which impoverished Americans testified to the difficulty of supplying nutritious meals to their families on limited incomes. But most of those who testified, as McGovern later recalled, were "vastly overweight." This led one senior senator on his committee to say to him, "George, this is ridiculous. These people aren't suffering from malnutrition. They're all overweight."

leisure time to exercise that rich people do; they don't have the money to join health clubs, and they live in neighborhoods without parks and sidewalks, so their kids don't have the opportunities to exercise and walk. These explanations may be true, but they stretch the imagination, and the contradiction gets still more glaring the deeper we delve.

If we look in the literature—which the experts have not in this case—we can find numerous populations that experienced levels of obesity similar to those in the United States, Europe, and elsewhere today but with no prosperity and few, if any, of the ingredients of Brownell's toxic environment: no cheeseburgers, soft drinks, or cheese curls, no drive-in windows, computers, or televisions (sometimes not even books, other than perhaps the Bible), and no overprotective mothers keeping their children from roaming free.

In these populations, incomes weren't rising; there were no labor-saving devices, no shifts toward less physically demanding work or more passive leisure pursuits. Rather, some of these populations were poor beyond our ability to imagine today. Dirt poor. These are the populations that the overeating hypothesis tells us should be as lean as can be, and yet they were not.

Remember Hilde Bruch's wondering about all those really fat children in the midst of the Great Depression? Well, this kind of observation isn't nearly as unusual as we might think. Consider a Native American tribe in Arizona known as the Pima. Today the Pima may have the highest incidence of obesity and diabetes in the United States. Their plight is often evoked as an example of what happens when a traditional culture runs afoul of the toxic environment of modern America. The Pima used to be hardworking farmers and hunters, so it is said, and now they're sedentary wage earners, like the rest of us, driving to the same fast-food restaurants, eating the same snacks, watching the same television shows, and getting fat and diabetic just like the rest of us, only more so. "As the typical American diet became more available on the [Pima's Gila River] reservation after the [Second World] war," according to the National Institutes of Health, "people became *more* overweight."

The italics in the quote are mine, because, you see, the Pima had a weight problem well before the Second World War and even before the First, back when there was nothing particularly toxic about their environment at all, or at least not as it would be described today. Between 1901 and 1905, two anthropologists independently studied the Pima, and both commented on how fat they were, particularly the women.

The first was Frank Russell, a young Harvard anthropologist, whose seminal report on the Pima was published in 1908. Russell noted that many of the older Pima "exhibit a degree of obesity that is in striking contrast with the 'tall and sinewy' Indian conventionalized in popular thought." He also took this picture of the Pima he called "Fat Louisa."

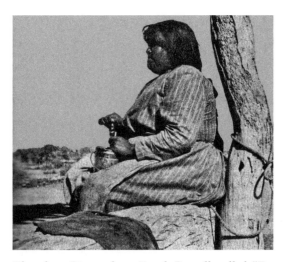

The obese Pima whom Frank Russell called "Fat Louisa" more than one hundred years ago surely didn't get fat because she ate at fast-food restaurants and watched too much television.

The second was Aleš Hrdlička, who was trained originally as a physician and would later serve as curator of physical anthropology at the Smithsonian Institution. Hrdlička visited the Pima in 1902 and again in 1905 as part of a series of expeditions he undertook to study the health and welfare of the native tribes of the region. "Especially well-nourished individuals, females and also males, occur in every tribe and at all ages," wrote Hrdlička about the Pima and nearby Southern Utes, "but real obesity is found almost exclusively among the Indians on reservations."

What makes this observation so remarkable is that the Pima, at the time, had just gone from being among the most affluent Native American tribes to among the poorest. Whatever made the Pima fat, prosperity and rising incomes had nothing to do with it; rather, the opposite seemed to be the case.

Through the 1850s, the Pima had been extraordinarily successful hunters and farmers. Game was abundant in the region, and the Pima were particularly adept at trapping it or killing it with bow and arrow. They also ate fish and clams from the Gila River, which ran through their territory. They raised corn, beans, wheat, melons, and figs on fields irrigated with Gila River water and raised cattle and chickens as well.

In 1846, when a U.S. Army battalion passed through Pima lands, John Griffin, the battalion's surgeon, described the Pima as "sprightly" and in "fine health" and noted that they also had "the greatest abundance of food"—storehouses full of it.* So much that when the California gold rush began three years later, the U.S government asked the Pima to provide food, and they did, to the tens of thousands of travelers who passed through their territory in the next decade, heading to California on the Sante Fe Trail.

*Griffin was not the only one to comment on the fine health and leanness of the Pima in the mid-nineteenth century. The women "have good figures, with full chests and finely formed limbs," wrote the U.S. boundary commissioner John Bartlett, for instance, in the summer of 1852; the men "are generally lean and lank, with very small limbs and narrow chests."

With the California gold rush, the relative paradise of the Pima came to an end and, with it, their affluence. Anglo-Americans and Mexicans began settling in large numbers in the region. These newcomers—"some of the vilest specimens of humanity that the white race has produced," wrote Russell—hunted the local game near to extinction, and diverted the Gila River water to irrigate their own fields at the expense of the Pimas'.

By the 1870s, the Pima were living through what they called the "years of famine." "The marvel is that the starvation, despair, and dissipation that resulted did not overwhelm the tribe," wrote Russell. When Russell and Hrdlička appeared, in the first years of the twentieth century, the tribe was still raising what crops it could but was now relying on government rations for day-to-day sustenance.

So why were they fat? Years of starvation are supposed to take weight off, not put it on or leave it on, as the case may be. And if the government rations were simply excessive, making the famines a thing of the past, then why would the Pima get fat on the abundant rations and not on the abundant food they'd had prior to the famines? Perhaps the answer lies in the type of food being consumed, a question of quality rather than quantity. This is what Russell was suggesting when he wrote that "certain articles of their food appear to be markedly flesh producing."

Hrdlička also thought that the Pima should be thin, considering the precarious state of their existence, and so he said, "The role played by food in the production of obesity among the Indians is apparently indirect." This left him leaning toward physical inactivity as the cause, or at least *relative* physical inactivity. In other words, the Pima might have been more active than we are today, considering the rigors of preindustrial agriculture, but they were sedentary in comparison with what they used to be. This is what Hrdlička called "the change from their past active life to the present state of not a little indolence." But then he couldn't explain why the women were typically the fat ones, even though these women did virtually all the hard labor in the villages—harvesting the crops, grinding the grain, even carrying the heavy burdens when the pack animals were unavailable. Hrdlička was also troubled by another local tribe, the Pueblo, who had "been of sedentary habits since ancient times" but weren't fat.

So maybe the culprit *was* the type of food. The Pima were already eating everything "that enters into the dietary of the white man," as Hrdlička said. This might have been key. The Pima diet in 1900 had characteristics very similar to the diets many of us are eating a century later, but not in quantity, in quality.

As it turns out, half a dozen trading posts had opened on the Pima reservation after 1850. From these, as the anthropologist Henry Dobyns has noted, the Pima bought "sugar, coffee and canned goods to replace traditional foodstuffs lost ever since whites had settled in their territory." Moreover, the great bulk of the government rations distributed to the reservations was white flour, as well as a significant amount of sugar, at least significant for the Pima of a century ago. These were quite likely the critical factors, as I will be arguing throughout this book.

If the Pima were the sole example of a population that was both very poor and beset by obesity, we could write them off as an exception to the rule—the single eyewitness whose testimony disagrees with copious others. But there were, as I said, numerous such populations, numerous witnesses to the presence of high levels of obesity in extremely poor populations. The Pima were the flag bearers in a parade of witnesses whose testimony never gets heard and who demonstrate that it's possible to become fat when you're poor, hardworking, and even underfed. Let's examine what they have to say, and then we'll move on.

A quarter-century after Russell and Hrdlička visited the Pima, two researchers from the University of Chicago studied another Native American tribe, the Sioux living on the South Dakota Crow Creek Reservation. These Sioux lived in shacks "unfit for occupancy," often four to eight family members per room. Many had no plumbing and no running water. Forty percent of the children lived in homes without any kind of toilets. Fifteen families, with thirty-two children among them, lived "chiefly on bread and coffee." This was poverty almost beyond our imagination today.

Yet their obesity rates were not much different from what we have today in the midst of our epidemic: 40 percent of the adult women on the reservation, more than a quarter of the men, and 10 percent of the children, according to the University of Chicago report, "would be termed distinctly fat." It could be argued that maybe their reservation life of what Hrdlička had called "not a little indolence" was causing their obesity, but the researchers noted another pertinent fact about these Sioux: one-fifth of the adult women, a quarter of the men, and a quarter of the children were "extremely thin."

The diets on the reservation, much of which, once again, came from government rations, were deficient in calories, as well as protein and essential vitamins and minerals. The impact of these dietary deficiencies was hard to miss: "Although no counts were taken, even a casual observer could not fail to note the great prevalence of decayed teeth, of bow legs, and of sore eyes and blindness among these families."

This combination of obesity and malnutrition or undernutrition (not enough calories) existing in the same populations is something that authorities today talk about as though it were a new phenomenon, but it's not. Here we have malnutrition or undernutrition coexisting with obesity in the same population eighty years ago. It's an important observation, and we'll see it again before we're done.

Let's look at several more examples:

1951: Naples, Italy

Ancel Keys, the University of Minnesota nutritionist almost singularly responsible for convincing us that the fat we eat and the cholesterol in our blood are causes of heart disease, visits Naples to study the diet and health of the Neapolitans.

"There is no mistaking the general picture"—he later writes—

"a little lean meat once or twice a week was the rule, butter was almost unknown, milk was never drunk except in coffee or for infants, 'colazione' [breakfast] on the job often meant half a loaf of bread crammed with baked lettuce or spinach. Pasta was eaten every day, usually also with bread (no spreads) and a fourth of the calories were provided by olive oil and wine. There was no evidence of nutritional deficiency *but the working-class women were fat.*"

What Keys didn't say was that most people in Naples and in fact all of southern Italy were exceedingly poor at the time. The Neapolitans had been devastated by the Second World War, so much so that a tragic sight during the latter years of the war was lines of mothers and housewives prostituting themselves to Allied soldiers to get money to feed their families. A postwar parliamentary inquiry portrayed the region as essentially a third-world nation. There was little meat to be had, which was why little meat was consumed, and malnutrition was common. Only by the late 1950s, long after Keys's visit, did reconstruction efforts begin to show any significant progress.

One other fact worth noting is how closely Keys's description of the Neapolitan diet matches the Mediterranean diet that is all the rage these days, even down to the copious olive oil and the red wine, or the grandmotherly diets that Michael Pollan recommends in *In Defense of Food:* "Eat food, not too much, mostly plants." Certainly these people were eating not too much. A 1951 survey ranked Italy and Greece as having less food available per capita than any other countries in Europe—twenty-four hundred calories daily, compared with thirty-eight hundred calories available per capita in the United States at that time. And yet "the working-class women were fat." Not the rich women but the ones who had to work hard for a living.

1954: The Pima Again

Bureau of Indian Affairs researchers weigh and measure the Pima children and report that more than half, boys and girls both, are obese by age eleven. Living conditions on the Gila River Reservation: "Widespread poverty."

1959: Charleston, South Carolina

Among African Americans, 18 percent of the men and 30 percent of the women are obese. Cash incomes for the heads of families range from $9 to $53 per week, or the equivalent of about $65 to $390 per week today.

1960: Durban, South Africa

Among Zulu, 40 percent of the adult women are obese. Women in their forties average 175 pounds. The women, on average, are twenty pounds *heavier* and four inches *shorter* than the men, but this does not mean they are better fed—excessive adiposity, the researchers report, is often accompanied by numerous signs of malnutrition.

1961: Nauru, the South Pacific

A local physician describes the situation bluntly: "By European standards, everyone past puberty is grossly overweight."

1961–63: Trinidad, West Indies

A team of nutritionists from the United States reports that malnutrition is a serious medical problem on the island, but so is obesity. Nearly a third of the women older than twenty-five are obese. The average caloric intake among these women is estimated at fewer than two thousand calories a day—*less than the minimum* recommended at the time by the Food and Agriculture Organization of the United Nations as necessary for a healthy diet.

1963: Chile

Obesity is described as "the main nutritional problem of Chilean adults." Twenty-two percent of military personnel and 32 percent of white-collar workers are obese. Among factory workers, 35 percent of males and 39 percent of females are obese. These factory workers are the most interesting, because their jobs quite likely involve significant physical labor.

1964–65: Johannesburg, South Africa

Researchers from the South African Institute for Medical Research study urban Bantu "pensioners" older than sixty—"the most indigent of elderly Bantu," which means the poorest members of an exceedingly poor population. The women in this population average 165 pounds. Thirty percent of them are "severely overweight." The average weight of "poor white" women is also reported to be 165 pounds.

1965: North Carolina

Twenty-nine percent of adult Cherokee on the Qualla Reservation are obese.

1969: Ghana

Twenty-five percent of the women and 7 percent of the men attending medical outpatient clinics in Accra are obese, including half of all women in their forties. "It may be reasonably concluded that severe obesity is common in women aged 30 to 60," writes an associate professor at the University of Ghana Medical School, and it is "fairly common knowledge that many market women in the coastal towns of West Africa are fat."

1970: Lagos, Nigeria

Five percent of the men are obese, as are nearly 30 percent of the women. Of women between fifty-five and sixty-five, 40 percent are very obese.

1971: Rarotonga, the South Pacific

Forty percent of the adult women are obese; 25 percent are "grossly obese."

1974: Kingston, Jamaica

Rolf Richards, a British-trained physician running a diabetes clinic at the University of the West Indies, reports that 10 percent of the adult men in Kingston and two-thirds of the women are obese.

1974: Chile (again)

A nutritionist from the Catholic University in Santiago reports on a study of thirty-three hundred factory workers, most engaged in heavy labor. "Only" 11 percent of the men and 9 percent of the women are "severely undernourished"; "only" 14 percent of the men and 15 percent of the women are "severely overweight." Of those forty-five and older, nearly 40 percent of the men and 50 percent of the women are obese. He also reports on studies in Chile from the 1960s, noting that "the lowest incidence [of obesity] exists among farm workers. Office workers show the most obesity, but it is also *common among slum dwellers.*"

1978: Oklahoma

Kelly West, the leading diabetes epidemiologist of the era, reports of the local Native American tribes that "men are very fat, women are even fatter."

1981–83: Starr County, Texas

On the Mexican border, two hundred miles south of San Antonio, William Mueller and colleagues from the University of Texas weigh and measure more than eleven hundred local Mexican-American residents. Forty percent of the men in their thirties are obese, although most of them are "employed in agricultural labor and/or work in the oil fields in the country." More than half the women in their fifties are obese. As for the living conditions, Mueller later describes them as "very simple. . . . There was one restaurant [in all of Starr County], a Mexican restaurant, and there was nothing else."

So why were they fat? What makes the overeating, calories-in/calories-out argument so convenient—suspiciously so—is that it always provides an answer to this question. If the population was so poor and malnourished that even the most stalwart believer in immoderate eating as the cause of obesity will have trouble imagining that they had too much food available—the Pima, for instance, in the 1900s or 1950s, the Sioux in the 1920s, the Trinidadians, or the slum dwellers of Chile in the 1960s and 1970s—then it can always be claimed that they must have been sedentary, or at least *too* sedentary. If they were obviously physically active—the Pima women, the Chilean factory workers, or the Mexican-American agricultural laborers and oil-field workers—then it can be claimed that they ate too much.

The same arguments can and will be made for individual cases as well. If we're fat and we can prove that we eat in moderation—we don't eat any more, say, than do our lean friends or siblings—the experts will confidently assume that we must be physically inactive. If we're carrying excess fat but obviously get plenty of exercise, then the experts will assume with equal confidence that we eat too much. If we're not gluttons, then we must be guilty of sloth. If we're not slothful, then gluttony is our sin.

These claims can be made (and often are) without knowing a single other pertinent fact about either the relevant populations or individuals. Indeed, they're often made with little desire or inclination to learn more.

In the early 1970s, nutritionists and research-minded physicians would discuss the observations of high levels of obesity in these poor populations, and they would occasionally do so with an open mind as to the cause. They were curious (as we should be) and hesitant to insist they knew the answer (as we should be).

This was a time when obesity was still considered a problem of "malnutrition" rather than "overnutrition," as it is today. A 1971 survey in Czechoslovakia, for instance, revealed that nearly 10 percent of the men were obese and a third of the women. When these data were reported in conference proceedings a few years later, the researcher who did so began with this statement: "Even a brief visit to Czechoslovakia would reveal that obesity is extremely common and that, as in other industrial countries, it is probably the most widespread form of *malnutrition*."

Referring to obesity as a "form of malnutrition" comes with no moral judgments attached, no belief system, no veiled insinuations of gluttony and sloth. It merely says that something is wrong with the food supply and it might behoove us to find out what.

Here's Rolf Richards, the British-turned-Jamaican diabetes specialist, discussing the evidence and the quandary of obesity and poverty in 1974, and doing so without any preconceptions: "It is difficult to explain the high frequency of obesity seen in a relatively impecunious [very poor] society such as exists in the West Indies, when compared to the standard of living enjoyed in the more developed countries. Malnutrition and subnutrition are common disorders in the first two years of life in these areas, and account for almost 25 per cent of all admissions to pediatric wards in Jamaica. Subnutrition continues in early childhood to the early teens. Obesity begins to manifest itself in the female population from the 25th year of life and reaches enormous proportions from 30 onwards."

When Richards says "subnutrition," he means there wasn't enough food. From birth through the early teens, West Indian children were exceptionally thin, and their growth was stunted. They needed more food, not just more nutritious food. Then obesity manifested itself, particularly among women, and exploded in these individuals as they reached maturity. This is the combination we saw among the Sioux in 1928 and later in Chile—malnutrition and/or undernutrition or subnutrition coexisting in the same population with obesity, often even in the same families.

Here's that same observation discussed more recently but now steeped in the paradigm that overeating is the cause of obesity. This is from a 2005 *New England Journal of Medicine* article, "A Nutrition Paradox—Underweight and Obesity in Developing Countries," written by Benjamin Caballero, head of the Center for Human Nutrition at Johns Hopkins University. Caballero describes his visit to a clinic in the slums of São Paulo, Brazil. The waiting room, he writes, was "full of mothers with thin, stunted young children, exhibiting the typical signs of chronic undernutrition. Their appearance, sadly, would surprise few who visit poor urban areas in the developing world. What might come as a surprise is that many of the mothers holding those under-nourished infants were themselves overweight."

Caballero then describes the difficulty that he believed this phenomenon presents: "The coexistence of underweight and overweight *poses a challenge to public health programs*, since the aims of programs to reduce undernutrition are obviously in conflict with those for obesity prevention." Put simply, if we want to prevent obesity, we have to get people to eat less, but if we want to prevent undernutrition, we have to make more food available. What do we do?

The italics in the Caballero quote are mine, not his. The coexistence of thin, stunted children, exhibiting the typical signs of chronic undernutrition, with mothers who are themselves overweight doesn't pose a challenge to public-health programs, as Caballero suggested; it poses a challenge to our beliefs—our paradigm.

If we believe that these mothers were overweight because they ate too much, and we know the children are thin and stunted because they're not getting enough food, then we're assuming that the mothers were consuming superfluous calories that they could have given to their children to allow them to thrive. In other words, the mothers are willing to starve their children so that they themselves can overeat. This goes against everything we know about maternal behavior.

So what's it going to be? Do we throw out everything we believe about maternal behavior so we can keep our beliefs about obesity and overeating intact? Or do we question our beliefs about the cause of obesity and let our beliefs about the sacrifices mothers will make for their children remain intact?

Again, the coexistence of underweight and overweight in the

same populations and even in the same families doesn't pose a challenge to public-health programs; it poses a challenge to our beliefs about the cause of obesity and overweight. And it shouldn't be the only thing that does, as we'll see in the chapters that follow.

2

The Elusive Benefits of Undereating

In the early 1990s, the National Institutes of Health set out to investigate a few critical issues of women's health. The result was the Women's Health Initiative (WHI), a collection of studies that would cost in the neighborhood of a billion dollars. Among the questions that the researchers hoped to answer was whether low-fat diets actually prevent heart disease or cancer, at least in women. So they enrolled nearly fifty thousand women in a trial, chose twenty thousand at random, and instructed them to eat a low-fat diet, rich in fruits, vegetables, and fiber. These women were given regular counseling to motivate them to stay on the diet.

One of the effects of this counseling, or maybe of the diet itself, is that the women also decided, consciously or unconsciously, to eat less. According to the WHI researchers, the women, on average, consumed 360 calories a day less on their diets than they did when they first agreed to participate. If we believe that obesity is caused by overeating, we might say that these women were "undereating" by 360 calories a day. They were eating almost 20 percent fewer calories than what public-health agencies tell us such women should be eating.

The result? After eight years of such undereating, these women lost an average of *two pounds* each. And their average waist circumference—a measure of abdominal fat—*increased*.

This suggests that whatever weight these women lost, if they did, was not fat but lean tissue — muscle.*

How is such a thing possible? If our weight is really determined by the difference between the calories we consume and the calories we expend, these women should have slimmed down significantly. A pound of fat contains roughly thirty-five hundred calories' worth of energy. If these women were really undereating by 360 calories every day, they should have lost more than two pounds of fat (seven thousand calories' worth) in the first three weeks, and more than thirty-six pounds in the first year.† And these women had plenty of fat to lose. Almost half began the study obese; the great majority were at the very least overweight.

One possibility, of course, is that the researchers failed miserably at assessing how much these women ate. Maybe the women deceived the investigators and themselves as well. Maybe they didn't undereat by 360 calories a day. "We have no idea what these women were really eating because, like most people when asked about their diet, they lied about it," as Michael Pollan suggested in *The New York Times*.

Another possibility is that this reduction in calories, this multiyear exercise in undereating, just didn't do what it was expected to do.

Of all the reasons to question the idea that overeating causes obesity, the most obvious has always been the fact that undereating doesn't cure it.

---

*This wasn't the only disappointing result in the study. The WHI investigators also reported that the low-fat diet failed to prevent heart disease, cancer, or anything else.

†This calculation is oversimplified to make a point. If it is corrected for the observation that subjects who lose weight in diet studies expend less energy as they do it, then the amount of weight loss expected with this energy deficit should be less: approximately 1.6 pounds at three weeks and twenty-two pounds at one year. I owe this correction to Kevin Hall, a biophysicist at the NIH, who points out that the corrected numbers are "still a far cry from the observed value!"

The Elusive Benefits of Undereating

Yes, it's true: If you are stranded on a desert island and starved for months on end, you will waste away, whether you're fat or thin to begin with. Even if you are just semi-starved, your fat will melt away, as will a good share of your muscle. Try the same prescription in the real world, though, and try to keep it up indefinitely — try to maintain the weight loss — and it works very rarely indeed, if at all.

This should come as no surprise. As I suggested earlier, with the assistance of Hilde Bruch's wisdom and experience, most of us who are fat spend much of our lives *trying* to eat less. If it doesn't work when the motivation is merely decades of the intense negative reinforcement that accompanies obesity — social ostracism, physical impairment, increased rate of disease — can we really expect it to work just because an authority figure in a white coat insists that we give it a try? The fat person who has never tried to undereat is a rare bird. If you're still fat, as Bruch noted, that's a good reason to assume that undereating failed to cure you of this particular affliction, even if it has some short-term success at treating the most conspicuous symptom — excess adiposity.

The very first time anyone published a review of the efficacy of undereating as a treatment for obesity — the psychologist Albert Stunkard and his colleague Mavis McLaren-Hume, in 1959 — this was their conclusion. Nothing much has changed since. Stunkard said their study was motivated by what he called the "paradox" between his own failure to treat obese patients successfully at his New York Hospital clinic by restricting how much they eat and "the widespread assumption that such treatment was easy and effective."

Stunkard and McLaren-Hume combed the medical literature and managed to find eight articles in which physicians reported on their success rates treating obese and overweight patients in their clinics. The results, said Stunkard, were "remarkably similar and remarkably poor." Most of these clinics were prescribing diets that allowed only eight hundred or one thousand calories a day — maybe half what the WHI women said they were eating — and still only one in four patients ever lost as much as twenty pounds;

only one in twenty patients managed to lose as much as forty pounds. Stunkard also reported on his own experience prescribing "balanced diets" of eight hundred to fifteen hundred calories a day to a hundred obese patients in his own clinic: only twelve lost as much as twenty pounds, and only one lost forty pounds. "Two years after the end of treatment," Stunkard wrote, "only two patients had maintained their weight loss."*

The more recent assessments benefit from the use of computers and elaborate statistical analyses, but the results, as Stunkard might say, are still remarkably similar and remarkably poor. Prescribing low-calorie diets for obese and overweight patients, according to a 2007 review from Tufts University, leads, at best, to "modest weight losses" that are "transient"—that is, temporary. Typically, nine or ten pounds are lost in the first six months. After a year, much of what was lost has been regained.

The Tufts review was an analysis of all the relevant diet trials in the medical journals since 1980. The single largest such trial ever done yields the very same answer.† The researchers were from Harvard and the Pennington Biomedical Research Center, which is in Baton Rouge, Louisiana, and is the most influential academic obesity-research institute in the United States. Together they enrolled more than eight hundred overweight and obese subjects and then randomly assigned them to eat one of four diets. These diets were marginally different in nutrient composition (proportions of protein, fat, and carbohydrates), but all were substantially the same in that the subjects were supposed to undereat by 750 calories a day, a significant amount. The subjects were also given "intensive behavioral counseling" to keep them on their diets, the kind of professional assistance that few of us

---

*Although Stunkard's analysis has widely been perceived as a condemnation of all methods of dietary treatment of obesity, the studies he reviewed included only calorie-restricted diets.

†I don't count the WHI low-fat diet trial, because that was aimed at preventing heart disease and cancer, not losing weight.

ever get when we try to lose weight. They were even given meal plans every two weeks to help them with the difficult chore of cooking tasty meals that were also sufficiently low in calories.

The subjects began the study, on average, fifty pounds overweight. They lost, on average, only nine pounds. And, once again, just as the Tufts review would have predicted, most of the nine pounds came off in the first six months, and most of the participants were gaining weight back after a year. No wonder obesity is so rarely cured. Eating less—that is, undereating—simply doesn't work for more than a few months, if that.

This reality, however, hasn't stopped the authorities from recommending the approach, which makes reading such recommendations an exercise in what psychologists call "cognitive dissonance," the tension that results from trying to hold two incompatible beliefs simultaneously.

Take, for instance, the *Handbook of Obesity*, a 1998 textbook edited by three of the most prominent authorities in the field— George Bray, Claude Bouchard, and W. P. T. James. "Dietary therapy remains the cornerstone of treatment and the reduction of energy intake continues to be the basis of successful weight reduction programs," the book says. But it then states, a few paragraphs later, that the results of such energy-reduced restricted diets "are known to be poor and not long-lasting." So why is such an ineffective therapy the cornerstone of treatment? The *Handbook of Obesity* neglects to say.

The latest edition (2005) of *Joslin's Diabetes Mellitus*, a highly respected textbook for physicians and researchers, is a more recent example of this cognitive dissonance. The chapter on obesity was written by Jeffrey Flier, an obesity researcher who is now dean of Harvard Medical School, and his wife and research colleague, Terry Maratos-Flier. The Fliers also describe "reduction of caloric intake" as "the cornerstone of any therapy for obesity." But then they enumerate all the ways in which this cornerstone fails. After examining approaches from the most subtle reductions in calories (eating, say, one hundred calories less each day with the hope of losing a pound every five weeks) to low-calorie diets of eight hundred to one thousand calories a day to very low-calorie diets (two hundred to six hundred calories) and even total starvation, they conclude that "none of these approaches has any proven merit." Alas.

Until the 1970s, low-calorie diets were referred to in medical literature as "semi-starvation" diets. After all, what's expected on these diets is that we eat half or even less of what we'd typically prefer to eat. But we can't be expected to semi-starve ourselves for more than a few months, let alone indefinitely, which is what such diets implicitly require if we are to maintain whatever weight loss we may initially experience. Very low-calorie diets are known as "fasts" because they allow barely any food at all. Again, it's hard to imagine fasting for more than a few weeks, maybe a month or two at best, and certainly we cannot keep it up forever once our excess fat is lost.

The two researchers who may have had the best track record in the world treating obesity in an academic setting were George Blackburn and Bruce Bistrian of Harvard Medical School. In the 1970s, they began treating obese patients with a six-hundred-calorie-a-day diet of only lean meat, fish, and fowl. They treated thousands of patients, said Bistrian. Half of them lost more than forty pounds. "This is an extraordinarily effective and safe way to get large amounts of weight loss," Bistrian said. But then Bistrian and Blackburn gave up on the therapy, because they didn't know what to tell their patients to do after the weight was lost. The patients couldn't be expected to live on six hundred calories a day forever, and if they returned to eating normally, they'd gain the weight right back. The only medically acceptable alternative, said Bistrian, was to give the patients drugs to kill their appetites, and they weren't willing to do that.

So, even if you lose most of your excess fat on one of these diets, you're then stuck with the what-happens-now problem. If you lose weight eating only six hundred calories a day, or even twelve hundred, should it come as a surprise that you get fat again when you return to eating two thousand calories a day or more? This is why the experts say a diet has to be something we can follow for life—a lifestyle program. But how is it possible to semi-starve ourselves or fast for more than a short time? As Bistrian said when I interviewed him a few years ago, echoing Bruch half a century earlier, undereating isn't a treatment or cure for obesity; it's a way of temporarily reducing the most obvious symptom. And if undereating isn't a treatment or a cure, this certainly suggests that overeating is not a cause.

3

The Elusive Benefits of Exercise

Imagine you're invited to a celebratory dinner. The chef's talent is legendary, and the invitation says that this particular dinner is going to be a feast of monumental proportions. Bring your appetite, you're told—come hungry. How would you do it?

You might try to eat less over the course of the day—maybe even skip lunch, or breakfast and lunch. You might go to the gym for a particularly vigorous workout, or go for a longer run or swim than usual, to work up an appetite. You might even decide to walk to the dinner, rather than drive, for the same reason.

Now let's think about this for a moment. The instructions that we're constantly being given to lose weight—eat less (decrease the calories we take in) and exercise more (increase the calories we expend)—are the very same things we'll do if our purpose is to make ourselves hungry, to build up an appetite, to eat more. Now the existence of an obesity epidemic coincident with half a century of advice to eat less and exercise more begins to look less paradoxical.*

We've seen the problems with eating less to produce weight loss. Now let's examine the flip side of the calories-in/calories-out equation. What happens when we increase our energy expenditure by upping our level of physical activity?

*Chris Williams, who blogs under the name Asclepius, had this insight.

It's now commonly believed that sedentary behavior is as much a cause of our weight problems as how much we eat. And because the likelihood that we'll get heart disease, diabetes, and cancer increases the fatter we become, the supposedly sedentary nature of our lives is now considered a causal factor in these diseases as well. Regular exercise is now seen as an essential means of prevention for all the chronic ailments of our day (except, of course, those of joints and muscles that are caused by excessive exercise).

Considering the ubiquity of the message, the hold it has on our lives, and the elegant simplicity of the notion—burn calories, lose weight, prevent disease—wouldn't it be nice if it were true? As a culture, we certainly believe it is. Faith in the health benefit of physical activity is now so deeply ingrained in our consciousness that it's often considered the one fact in the controversial science of health and lifestyle that must never be questioned.

There are indeed excellent reasons to exercise regularly. We can increase our endurance and fitness by doing so; we may live longer, perhaps, as the experts suggest, by reducing our risk of heart disease or diabetes. (Although this has yet to be rigorously tested.) We may simply feel better about ourselves, and it's quite clear that many of us who do exercise regularly, as I do, become exceedingly fond of the activity. But the question I want to explore here is not whether exercise is fun or good for us (whatever that ultimately means) or a necessary adjunct of a healthy lifestyle, as the authorities are constantly telling us, but whether it will help us maintain our weight if we're lean, or lose weight if we're not.

The answer appears to be no.

Let's look at the evidence. I want to begin with the observation I made in chapter 1 that obesity associates with poverty. In the United States, Europe, and other developed nations, the poorer people are, the fatter they're likely to be. It's also true that the poorer we are, the more likely we are to work at physically demanding occupations, to earn our living with our bodies rather than our brains.

It's the poor and disadvantaged who do the grunt work of

developed nations, who sweat out a living not just figuratively but literally. They may not belong to health clubs or spend their leisure time (should they have any) training for their next marathon, but they're far more likely than those more affluent to work in the fields and in factories, as domestics and gardeners, in the mines and on construction sites. That the poorer we are the fatter we're likely to be is one very good reason to doubt the assertion that the amount of energy we expend on a day-to-day basis has any relation to whether we get fat. If factory workers can be obese, as I discussed earlier, and oil-field laborers, it's hard to imagine that the day-to-day expenditure of energy makes much of a difference.

Another very good reason to doubt that assertion is, once again, the obesity epidemic itself. We've been getting steadily fatter for the past few decades, and this might suggest, as many authorities do—the World Health Organization among them— that we've been getting more sedentary. But the evidence suggests the opposite, certainly in the United States, where the obesity epidemic has coincided with what we might call an epidemic of leisure-time physical activity, of health clubs and innovative means of expending energy (in-line skating, mountain biking, step and elliptical machines, spinning and aerobics, Brazilian martial-arts classes—the list goes on), virtually all of which were either invented or radically redesigned since the obesity epidemic began.*

Until the 1970s, Americans were not believers in the need to spend leisure hours sweating, not if they could avoid it. In the mid-1970s, as was pointed out by William Bennett and Joel Gurin in their 1982 book on obesity, *The Dieter's Dilemma*, it "still

---

*There are many ways to quantify this epidemic of physical activity. Health-club industry revenues, for example, increased from an estimated $200 million in 1972 to $16 billion in 2005—a seventeen-fold increase when adjusted for inflation. The first year that the Boston Marathon had more than 300 entrants was 1964; in 2009, more than 26,000 men and women ran. The first New York City

seemed a little strange to see people go running down a city street in the colorful equivalent of underwear." But this is no longer the case. Indeed, *The New York Times* reported in 1977 that the United States was *then* in the midst of an "exercise explosion," and this was only happening because the widespread belief of the 1960s that exercise was "bad for you" had been transformed into the "new conventional wisdom—that strenuous exercise is good for you." In 1980, *The Washington Post* reported that one hundred million Americans had become active members of the "new fitness revolution" and that many of these "would have been derided as 'health nuts' " just a decade earlier. "What we are seeing," the *Post* reported, "is one of the late twentieth century's major sociological events."

But if sedentary behavior makes us fat and physical activity prevents it, shouldn't the "exercise explosion" and the "new fitness revolution" have launched an epidemic of leanness rather than coinciding with an epidemic of obesity?

As it turns out, very little evidence exists to support the belief that the number of calories we expend has any effect on how fat we are. In August 2007, the American Heart Association (AHA) and the American College of Sports Medicine (ACSM) addressed this evidence in a particularly damning manner when they published joint guidelines on physical activity and health. The ten expert authors included many of the preeminent proponents of the essential role of exercise in a healthy lifestyle. Put simply, these were people who really want us to exercise and might be tempted to stack the evidence in favor of our doing so. Thirty minutes of

Marathon was in 1970, with 137 entrants; in 1980, there were 16,000 official runners; and in 2008, 39,000, although nearly 60,000 applied. According to the website MarathonGuide.com, nearly 400 marathons were scheduled in the United States in 2009, not to mention countless half-marathons, more than 50 ultramarathons (100 miles long), and 160-plus other "ultras" (up to 3,100 miles).

moderately vigorous physical activity, they said, five days a week, was necessary to "maintain and promote health."

But when it came to the question of how exercising affects our getting fat or staying lean, these experts could only say: "It is reasonable to assume that persons with relatively high daily energy expenditures would be less likely to gain weight over time, compared with those who have low energy expenditures. So far, data to support this hypothesis are not particularly compelling."

The AHA/ACSM guidelines were a departure from the recent guidelines of other authoritative agencies—the U.S. Department of Agriculture (USDA), the International Association for the Study of Obesity, and the International Obesity Taskforce—all of which recommended that we should exercise an hour a day. But the reason these other authorities advocate more exercise is not to help us lose fat, which they tacitly acknowledge cannot be done by exercising alone; rather, it's to help us avoid getting fatter.

The logic behind the one-hour recommendations is based precisely on the paucity of evidence to support the notion that exercising any less has any effect. Since few studies exist to tell us what happens when people exercise for more than sixty minutes each day, these authorities can imagine that this much exercise *might* make a difference. The USDA guidelines have suggested that up to ninety minutes a day of moderately vigorous exercise— an hour and a half every day!—may be necessary just to *maintain* weight loss, but they have not suggested that weight can be lost by exercising more than ninety minutes.

The evidence leaves little room for argument. To call it "not particularly compelling," as the American Heart Association and the American College of Sports Medicine did, is, well, a little unduly generous. A report that these expert guidelines often defer to as the basis for their assessments was published in 2000 by two Finnish exercise physiologists. These researchers looked at the results of the dozen best-constructed experimental trials that addressed weight maintenance—that is, successful dieters who were trying to keep off the pounds they had shed. They found that everyone in these studies regained weight. Depending on the type of trial, exercise would either decrease the rate of that gain (by 3.2 ounces per month) or increase its rate (by 1.8 ounces). As the Finns themselves concluded, with characteristic understatement, the relationship between exercise and weight is "more complex" than they might otherwise have imagined.

One study that the Finns could not consider, because it was published in 2006, six years later, is particularly revealing, both in what it concluded and how those conclusions were interpreted. The authors were Paul Williams, a statistics expert at the Lawrence Berkeley National Laboratory in Berkeley, California, and Peter Wood, a Stanford University researcher who has been studying the effect of exercise on health since the 1970s. Williams and Wood collected detailed information on almost thirteen thousand habitual runners (all subscribers to *Runner's World* magazine) and then compared the weekly mileage of these runners with how much they weighed from year to year. Those who ran the most tended to weigh the least, but *all* these runners tended to get fatter with each passing year, even those who ran more than forty miles a week—eight miles a day, say, five days a week.

This observation led Williams and Wood, both believers in the doctrine of calories-in/calories-out, to suggest that even the most dedicated runners had to increase their distance by a few miles a week, year after year—expend even more energy as they got older—if they wanted to remain lean. If men added two miles to their weekly distance every year, and women three, according to Williams and Wood, then they *might* manage to remain lean, because this might mean expending in running the calories that they seemed fated otherwise to accumulate as fat.

Let's see where that logic takes us. Imagine a man in his twenties who runs twenty miles a week—say, four miles a day, five days a week. According to Williams and Wood (and the logic and mathematics of calories-in/calories-out), he will have to double that in his thirties (eight miles a day, five days a week) and triple it in his forties (twelve miles a day, five days a week) to keep fat from accumulating. A woman in her twenties who runs three miles a day, five times a week—an impressive but not excessive amount—would have to up her daily distance to fifteen miles in her forties to retain her youthful figure. If she does eight-minute miles, a nice pace for such a distance, she'd better be prepared to spend two hours on each of her running days to keep her weight in check.

If we believe in calories-in/calories-out, and that in turn leads us to conclude that we have to run half-marathons five days a week (in our forties, and more in our fifties, and more in our sixties . . .) to maintain our weight, it may, once again, be time to question our underlying beliefs. Maybe it's something other than the calories we consume and expend that determines whether we get fat.

The ubiquitous faith in the belief that the more calories we expend, the less we'll weigh is based ultimately on one observation and one assumption. The observation is that people who are lean tend to be more physically active than those of us who aren't. This is undisputed. Marathon runners as a rule are not overweight or obese; the front-runners in marathons often look emaciated.

But this observation tells us nothing about whether runners would be fatter if they didn't run or if the pursuit of distance running as a full-time hobby will turn a fat man or woman into a lean marathoner.

We base our belief in the fat-burning properties of exercise on the assumption that we can increase our energy expenditure (calories-out) without being compelled to increase our energy intake (calories-in). Burn 150 extra calories every day in exercise and keep it up for a month, as *New York Times* reporter Gina Kolata calculated in her 2004 book, *Ultimate Fitness*, and you could lose a pound "if you do not change your diet."

The key question, though, is whether this is a reasonable possibility. Is it true that we can increase our expenditure of calories, burn an extra 150 calories a day, say, or go from being sedentary to active or from active to very active, without changing our diet—without eating more—and without maybe decreasing the amount of energy we expend in the hours between our bouts of exercise?

The simple answer, again, is no. I've already introduced the concept that explains why, one that used to seem perfectly obvious but has now been relegated to the dustbin of exercise and nutrition history. This is the idea that if we increase our physical activity we will "work up an appetite." If you go for a walk or rake some leaves, take a long hike, play two sets of tennis or eighteen holes of golf, you work up an appetite. You get hungry or hungrier. Increase the energy you expend and the evidence is very good that you will increase the calories you consume to compensate.

That we have gotten to the place in our lives, and in the science of exercise, nutrition, and weight, where this concept of working up an appetite, of the body's increasing its intake of energy to compensate for its increased expenditure, has been forgotten is one of the stranger stories in the history of modern medical research, or at least I hope it is.

Until the 1960s, most clinicians who treated obese patients dismissed as naïve the notion that we could lose weight through exercise or gain it by being sedentary. When Russell Wilder, an obesity and diabetes specialist at the Mayo Clinic, lectured on obesity in 1932, he said his fat patients lost more weight with bed rest, "while unusually strenuous physical exercise slows the rate of loss." "The patient reasons quite correctly," Wilder said, "that the more exercise he takes the more fat should be burned and that loss of weight should be in proportion and he is discouraged to find that the scales reveal no progress."

The patient's reasoning had two flaws, as Wilder's contemporaries would point out. First, we burn surprisingly few calories doing moderate exercise, and, second, the effort can be easily undone, and probably will be, by mindless changes in diet. A 250-pound man will burn *three* extra calories climbing one flight of stairs, as Louis Newburgh of the University of Michigan calculated in 1942. "He will have to climb twenty flights of stairs to rid himself of the energy contained in one slice of bread!"

So why not skip the stairs and skip the bread and call it a day? After all, what are the chances that if a 250-pounder does climb twenty extra flights a day he won't eat the equivalent of an extra slice of bread before the day is done?

Yes, more strenuous exercise will burn more calories—"it really is much more effective to exercise hard enough to sweat," Kolata tells us, "and that is the only way to burn large numbers of calories"—but, as these physicians argued, it will also make you hungrier still.

"Vigorous muscle exercise usually results in immediate demand for a large meal," noted Hugo Rony of Northwestern University in 1940. "Consistently high or low energy expenditures result in consistently high or low levels of appetite. Thus men doing heavy physical work spontaneously eat more than men engaged in sedentary occupations. Statistics show that the average daily caloric intake of lumberjacks is more than 5,000 calories while that of tailors is only about 2,500 calories. Persons who change their occupation from light to heavy work or *vice versa* soon develop corresponding changes in their appetite." So, if a tailor becomes a lumberjack and, by doing so, takes to eating like one, why assume the same thing wouldn't happen, albeit to a lesser extent, to an overweight tailor who chooses to work out like a lumberjack for an hour a day?*

---

*When researchers now discuss the relationship between physical activity and calorie intake in populations, as opposed to individuals, this is still perceived as a given: as Walter Willett and Meir Stampfer of Harvard noted in the 1998 textbook *Nutritional Epidemiology:* "In most instances, energy intake can be interpreted as a crude measure of physical activity."

The dubious credit for why we came to believe otherwise goes almost exclusively to one man, Jean Mayer, who began his professional career at Harvard in 1950, proceeded to become the most influential nutritionist in the United States, and then, for sixteen years, served as president of Tufts University (where there is now a Jean Mayer USDA Human Nutrition Research Center on Aging). Those who have ever believed that they can lose fat and keep it off by exercising have Jean Mayer to thank.

As an authority on human weight regulation, Mayer was among the very first of a new breed, a type that has since come to dominate the field. His predecessors—Bruch, Wilder, Rony, Newburgh, and others—had all been physicians who worked closely with obese and overweight patients. Mayer was not. His training was in physiological chemistry; he wrote his doctoral thesis at Yale University on the relationship of vitamins A and C in rats. He would eventually publish hundreds of papers on nutrition, including why we get fat, but his job never actually required that he reduce a fat person to a healthy weight, and so his ideas were less fettered by real-life experience.

It was Mayer who pioneered the now ubiquitous practice of implicating sedentary living as the "most important factor" leading to obesity and the chronic diseases that accompany it. Modern Americans, said Mayer, were inert compared with their "pioneer forebears," who were "constantly engaged in hard physical labor." Every modern convenience, by this logic, from riding lawn mowers to the electric toothbrush, only serves to reduce the calories we expend. "The development of obesity," Mayer wrote in 1968, "is to a large extent the result of the lack of foresight of a civilization which spends tens of billions annually on cars, but is unwilling to include a swimming pool and tennis courts in the plans of every high school."

Mayer actually began extolling exercise as a means of weight control in the early 1950s, a few years out of graduate school, after studying a strain of obese mice that had a surprisingly small appetite. This seemed to absolve eating too much from being the cause of their obesity, so Mayer naturally assumed their sedentary behavior must be responsible, and they were certainly sedentary. They barely moved. By 1959, *The New York Times* was giving Mayer credit for having "debunked" the "popular theories" that exercise was of little value in weight control, which he hadn't.

Mayer acknowledged that appetite tended to increase with physical activity, but the heart of his argument was that it wasn't "necessarily" the case. He believed there was a loophole in the relationship between expending more energy and eating more as a result. "If exercise is decreased below a certain point," Mayer explained in 1961, "food intake no longer decreases. In other words, walking one-half hour a day may be equivalent to only four slices of bread,* but if you don't walk the half hour, you still want to eat the four slices." So, if you're sufficiently sedentary, you're going to eat just as much as you would if you were a little active and expended more energy.

Mayer based this conclusion on two (and only two) of his own studies from the mid-1950s.

The first was on laboratory rats, purporting to demonstrate that when these rats were forced to exercise for a few hours every day, they ate less than rats that didn't exercise at all. Mayer didn't say that they actually weighed less, only that they ate less. As it turns out, rats on these exercise programs eat more on days when they aren't forced to run and will expend less energy when they're not exercising. Their weights, however, remain the same as those of sedentary rats. And when rats are retired from these exercise programs, they eat more than ever and gain weight with age more rapidly than rats that are allowed to remain sedentary. With hamsters and gerbils, exercise increases body weight and body fat percentage. So exercising makes these particular rodents fatter, not leaner.

---

*Mayer was exaggerating to make his point. He often did.

The Elusive Benefits of Exercise

Mayer's second study was an assessment of the diet, physical activity, and weight of workers and merchants at a mill in West Bengal, India. This article is still cited—by the Institute of Medicine, for instance—as perhaps the only existing evidence that physical activity and appetite do not necessarily go hand in hand. But it, too, would never be replicated, despite (or perhaps because of) a half-century of improvements in methods of assessing diet and energy expenditure in humans.*

It helped that Mayer promoted his pro-exercise message with a fervor akin to a moral crusade. And as Mayer's political influence grew through the 1960s, this contributed to the appearance that his faith in the weight-reducing benefits of exercise was widely shared. In 1966, when the U.S. Public Health Service first advocated dieting *and* increased physical activity as the keys to weight loss, Mayer wrote the report. Three years later, he chaired a White House Conference on Food, Nutrition and Health. "The successful treatment of obesity must involve far reaching changes in life style," the conference report concluded. "These changes include alterations of dietary patterns and physical activity." In 1972, when Mayer began writing a syndicated newspaper column on nutrition, he came across like a diet doctor selling a patent claim. Exercise, he wrote, would "make weight melt away faster," and, "contrary to popular belief, exercise won't stimulate your appetite."

---

*The Bengali research is a case study in how bad supposedly seminal research can be in the field of nutrition. The jobs of the men working in this Indian mill, as Mayer reported, ranged from "extraordinarily inert" stall holders "who sat at their shop all day long" to furnace tenders who "shoveled ashes and coal" for a living. The evidence reported in Mayer's paper could have been used to demonstrate *any* point. The more active workers in the mill, for example, both weighed more *and* ate more than less active workers. As for the sedentary workers, the more sedentary they were, the *more* they ate, the *less* they weighed. The clerks who lived on the premises and sat all day long weighed ten to fifteen pounds *less* and were reported to have eaten four hundred calories *more* on average than clerks who had to walk three to six miles to work—or even than those clerks who walked to work and also played soccer every day.

Meanwhile, the evidence never supported Mayer's hypothesis—not in animals, as I said, and certainly not in humans. One remarkable study of the effect of physical activity on weight loss was published in 1989 by a team of Danish researchers. The Danes actually did train sedentary subjects to run marathons (26.2 miles). After eighteen months of training, and after actually running a marathon, the eighteen men in the study had lost an average of five pounds of body fat. As for the nine women subjects, the Danes reported, "no change in body composition was observed." That same year, Xavier Pi-Sunyer, director of the St. Luke's–Roosevelt Hospital Obesity Research Center in New York, reviewed the existing trials testing the notion that increasing exercise would lead to weight loss. His conclusion was identical to that of the Finnish review in 2000: "Decreases, increases, and no changes in body weight and body composition have been observed."

We bought into the idea that we could exercise more and not compensate by eating more because the health reporters bought it, and their articles in the lay press were widely read. The research literature itself was not.

In 1977, for instance, in the midst of the exercise explosion, the National Institutes of Health hosted its second ever conference on obesity and weight control, and the assembled experts concluded that "the importance of exercise in weight control is less than might be believed, because increases in energy expenditure due to exercise also tend to increase food consumption, and it is not possible to predict whether the increased caloric output will be outweighed by the greater food intake." That same year, the *New York Times Magazine* reported that there was "now strong evidence that regular exercise can and does result in substantial and—so long as the exercise is continued—permanent weight loss."*

By 1983, Jane Brody, personal-health reporter for the *Times*,

---

*That evidence was the "carefully controlled experiments" of Jean Mayer showing "that moderate amounts of exercise actually suppress appetite slightly."

was counting the numerous ways that exercise was "the key" to successful weight loss. By 1989, the same year Pi-Sunyer gave his pessimistic assessment of the actual evidence, *Newsweek* declared exercise an "essential" element of any weight-loss program. Now, according to the *Times*, on those infrequent occasions "when exercise isn't enough" to induce sufficient weight loss, "you must also make sure you don't overeat."

Why the obesity researchers and public-health authorities eventually came to believe this story is a different question. Umberto Eco offered a likely answer in his novel *Foucault's Pendulum*. "I believe that you can reach the point," Eco wrote, "where there is no longer any difference between developing the habit of pretending to believe and developing the habit of believing."

From the late 1970s onward, the primary factor fueling the belief that we can maintain or lose weight through exercise seemed to be the researchers' desire to believe it was true and their reluctance to acknowledge otherwise publicly. Although one couldn't help being "underwhelmed" by the actual evidence, as Judith Stern, Mayer's former student, wrote in 1986, it would be "shortsighted" to say that exercise was ineffective, because it meant ignoring the *possible* contributions of exercise to the prevention of obesity and to the maintenance of any weight loss that might have been induced by diet. These, of course, had never been demonstrated, either.

This philosophy came to dominate even the scientific discussions of exercise and weight, but it couldn't be reconciled with the simple notion that appetite and the amount we eat can be expected to increase the more we exercise. And so the idea of working up an appetite was jettisoned along the way. Physicians, researchers, exercise physiologists, even personal trainers at the gym took to thinking about hunger as though it were something that existed only in the brain, a question of willpower (whatever that is), not the natural consequence of a body's effort to get back the energy it has expended.

As for the researchers themselves, they invariably found a way to write their articles and reviews that allowed them to continue to promote exercise and physical activity, regardless of what the evidence actually showed. One common method was (and still is) to discuss only the results that seem to support the belief that physical activity and energy expenditure can determine how fat we are, while simply ignoring the evidence that refutes the notion, even if the latter is in much more plentiful supply.

Two experts in the *Handbook of Obesity*, for instance, reported as a reason to exercise that the Danish attempt to turn sedentary subjects into marathon runners had resulted in a loss of five pounds of body fat in male subjects; they neglected to mention, however, that it had zero influence on the women in the trial, which could be taken as a strong incentive not to exercise. (If your goal is to lose weight—even if your health and your life depend on it, as they very well may—would you train to run a twenty-six-mile foot race upon being told that you *might* lose five pounds of fat after a year and half of work?)

Other experts took to arguing that we could lose weight by weightlifting or resistance training rather than the kind of aerobic activity, like running, that was aimed purely at increasing our expenditure of calories. The idea here was that we could build muscle and lose fat, and so we'd be fitter even if our weight remained constant, because of the trade-off. Then the extra muscle would contribute to maintaining the fat loss, because it would burn off more calories—muscle being more metabolically active than fat.

To make this argument, though, these experts invariably ignored the actual numbers, because they, too, are unimpressive. If we replace five pounds of fat with five pounds of muscle, which is a significant achievement for most adults, we will increase our energy expenditure by two dozen calories a day. Once again, we're talking about the caloric equivalent of a quarter-slice of bread, with no guarantee that we won't be two-dozen-calories-a-day hungrier because of this. And once again we're back to the notion that it might be easier just to skip both the bread and the weightlifting.

Before I finish this discussion of exercise and energy expenditure, I want to return briefly to the guidelines published in August 2007 by the American Heart Association and the American College of Sports Medicine. "It is reasonable to assume that persons with relatively high daily energy expenditures would be less likely to gain weight over time, compared with those who have low energy expenditures," the expert authors had written. "So far, data to support this hypothesis are not particularly compelling."

Damaging as this may be to the notion that we can lose weight by exercising, the authors were unwilling to be definitive. They had slipped in a qualification, the words "so far." By doing so, they were leaving the door of possibility open. Maybe somebody, someday, would show scientifically that what these experts believed in their hearts to be true really was.

But they missed the point with their qualification. Here it is: this idea that we get fat because we're sedentary and we can get lean or prevent ourselves from fattening further by upping our energy expenditure is at least a century old. One of the most influential European authorities on obesity and diabetes, Carl von Noorden, suggested this in 1907. We can, in fact, trace it to the 1860s, when the obese British undertaker William Banting discussed his numerous failed attempts to lose weight in his best-selling *Letter on Corpulence*. A physician friend, wrote Banting, suggested he slim down by "increased bodily exertion." So Banting took up rowing "for a couple of hours in the early morning." He gained muscular vigor, he wrote, "but with it a prodigious appetite, which I was compelled to indulge, and consequently increased in weight, until my kind old friend advised me to forsake the exercise."

The experts from the AHA and the ACSM would like to think that maybe if we just put further effort into studying the relationship between exercise and weight—if we do the experiments in just the right ways—we will finally confirm what von Noorden and Banting's physician friend and a century of researchers and physicians and exercise aficionados ever since have argued somehow must be true.

The history of science suggests another interpretation: if people have been thinking about this idea for more than a century and trying to test it for decades and they still can't generate compelling evidence that it's true, it's probably not. We can't say it's not with absolute certainty, because science doesn't work that way. But we can say that there's now an exceedingly good chance it's simply wrong, one of the many seemingly reasonable ideas in the history of science that never panned out. And if reducing calories-in doesn't make us lose weight, and if increasing calories-out doesn't even prevent us from gaining it, maybe we should rethink the whole thing and find out what does.

4

The Significance
of Twenty Calories a Day

Twenty calories.

Next time someone tells us, as the World Health Organization does on its website, that the way to prevent "the burden of obesity" is "to achieve energy balance and a healthy weight," this is the number that should come immediately to mind. Next time we're told, as the U.S. Department of Agriculture tells us, that "to prevent gradual weight gain over time" all we need do is "make small decreases in food and beverage calories and increase physical activity," remember this number.

If either of these official declarations about weight were true, then the obesity problem would be a figment of our collective imaginations, not the most pressing public health issue of our age.

Weight gain is a gradual process, as the USDA suggests. Once you notice that you're putting on weight, as the logic of calories-in/calories-out dictates, you can make the appropriate small decreases in calories consumed, and increases in physical activity and all should be well again. You can skip a snack here and a dessert there; you can walk more, spend a few extra minutes at the gym, and that should do it. Even if you put on ten pounds before you notice the difference, you know what's necessary to take them off.

So why doesn't that work? Why is there obesity at all, and why is its cure rate so dismally low, if all that's necessary to prevent it is to undo the positive caloric balance, the overeating, that allegedly causes it?

This is where the twenty calories come in. A pound of fat contains about thirty-five hundred calories' worth of energy. This is why nutritionists tell us that losing a pound a week requires that we create an average energy deficit of five hundred calories a day—five hundred calories times seven days equals thirty-five hundred calories a week.*

Now let's look at the math from the perspective of weight gain rather than weight loss. How many calories do we have to overeat daily to accumulate two new pounds of fat every year—fifty pounds in a quarter-century? How many calories do we have to consume but not expend, stashing them away in our fat tissue, to transform ourselves, as many of us do, from lean twenty-five-year-olds to obese fifty-year-olds?

Twenty calories a day.

Twenty calories a day times the 365 days in a year comes to a little more than seven thousand calories stored as fat every year—two pounds of excess fat.

If it were true that our adiposity is determined by calories-in/calories-out, then this is one implication: you only need to overeat, on average, by twenty calories a day to gain fifty extra pounds of fat in twenty years. You need only to rein yourself in by this amount—undereat by twenty calories a day—to undo it.

Twenty calories is less than a single bite of a McDonald's hamburger or a croissant. It's less than two ounces of Coke or Pepsi or the typical beer. Less than three potato chips. Maybe three small bites of an apple. In short, not very much at all.

Twenty calories is less than 1 percent of the daily caloric intake that the U.S. National Academy of Sciences has recommended

---

*Once again, this is vastly oversimplified, and it doesn't work in practice, but the arithmetic is right, and this is how the authorities perceive it. That's all we need to know at the moment.

for a middle-aged woman whose idea of regular physical activity is cooking and sewing; it's less than half a percent of the daily quota of calories recommended for an equally sedentary middle-aged man. That it's such an insignificant amount is what makes it so telling about the calories-in/calories-out idea. If what's necessary "to maintain weight," as the National Institutes of Health says, is to "balance the energy we eat with the energy we use," then consuming an average of twenty calories a day more than you expend, according to the logic of calories-in/calories-out, will eventually make you obese.

Ask yourself: How is it possible that anyone stays lean, if all it takes to grow gradually obese is to overshoot this point of energy balance by twenty calories daily? Because quite a few people do stay lean. And, in fact, even those who are overweight or obese manage to maintain their weight, heavy as they may be, for years and decades. They may be fat, but they are still balancing the calories they take in with the calories they expend, apparently, to better than that twenty-calories-a-day average, because they are not getting fatter still. How do they do that?

One or two bites or swallows too many (out of the hundred or two we might take to consume a day's worth of sustenance) and we're doomed. If the difference between eating not too much and eating too much is less than a hundredth of the total amount of calories we consume, and that in turn has to be matched with our energy expenditure, to which we are, for the most part, completely in the dark, how can anyone possibly eat with such accuracy? To put it simply, the question we should be asking is not why some of us get fat, but how any of us avoids this fate.

This is a question that researchers asked in the first half of the twentieth century with regard to this arithmetic, back before calories-in/calories-out became the conventional wisdom. In 1936, Eugene Du Bois of Cornell University, then considered the leading U.S. authority on nutrition and metabolism, calculated that a 165-pound man who manages to maintain his weight for two decades—to gain no more than two pounds during those twenty years—is matching his calories-in to his calories-out to within a twentieth of 1 percent, "an exactness," Du Bois wrote, "which is equaled by few mechanical devices."

"We do not yet know why certain individuals grow fat," Du Bois wrote. "Perhaps it would be more accurate to say that we do not know why all the individuals in this over-nourished community do not grow fat." Considering the accuracy required to maintain a stable weight, he added, "there is no stranger phenomena than the maintenance of a constant body weight under marked variation in bodily activity and food consumption."

The fact that many people do remain lean for decades (although it's less common now than in Du Bois's day), and that even those who are fat don't continuously get fatter, suggests there is something more going on with this business of weight regulation than can be explained by the notion that it's all about calories.

Let's consider some possibilities. Perhaps we maintain energy balance, say, by watching the scale or attending to the other signs of increasing adiposity and then adjusting our eating accordingly. This was one idea taken seriously by the experts in the 1970s: *Uh-oh, belt's too tight, getting fat again, better eat less.*

But animals obviously don't do that, and there's no reason to think that calories-in/calories-out doesn't apply to them as well. Yet species that begin their adult lives lean (leaving out of the discussion, for the moment, those that don't, such as walruses and hippopotami) remain lean with little apparent effort. How do they do it?

Maybe the only way to stay lean is to stay hungry—not terribly hungry but at least a little hungry. If we always leave a little on the plate, remain a tad unsatisfied, then we can be confident that our accumulated errors will fall on the side of eating too little rather than too much. Better to eat a few hundred calories less than we'd like than twenty calories more every day than we need. So either we live in a world where we rarely have enough food available or we consciously eat in moderation, which means pushing away from the table (or, for animals, walking away from the latest kill or cutting short a graze) before we're satiated.

But if eating in moderation means we consciously err on the side of too little food, why don't we all end up so lean that we appear emaciated? The arithmetic of calories-in/calories-out doesn't differentiate between losing and gaining weight; it says only that we must match calories consumed to calories expended. And if it's simply the case that lean populations are only those populations that don't have enough food available to overeat (by twenty calories, on average, every day), why is it that populations in this situation—like the ones we discussed earlier in which the children are thin and stunted and exhibit "the typical signs of chronic undernutrition"—can still have plenty of obese adults?

Surely something else is determining whether we gain fat or lose it, not just the conscious or unconscious balancing act of matching calories consumed and expended. I'll get to that in time. First I want to discuss what calories-in/calories-out has to say (or doesn't) about where we get fat, when we get fat, and why some people and animals don't.

5

Why Me? Why There? Why Then?

We typically talk about body fat as though either we have it to excess or we don't, a yes-or-no proposition. But this is an oversimplification of a far more complex phenomenon. Where on our bodies we get fat, and even when it happens, are important questions as well. The experts acknowledge this implicitly when they tell us that abdominal obesity (excessive belly fat) goes along with an increased risk for heart disease, but being fat on the hips or butt does not. That two people overate and so consumed more calories than they expended, though, tells us nothing about why their fat distribution might be so different and, with it, their risk of dying a premature death.

Why do some of us have double chins and others don't? How about fat ankles? Love handles? Why do some women have voluptuous accumulations of fat in their breasts and others little? How about big butts? The African women who have the prominent gluteal fat deposits known as "steatopygia," considered a sign of beauty in these populations, probably did not develop them by eating too much or exercising too little.

And if they didn't, why assume that these are acceptable explanations for the fat that we might be amassing on our own rear ends?

Before the Second World War, the physicians who studied obesity believed that much could be explained by observing how fat was distributed on their obese patients. Putting photos of these sub-

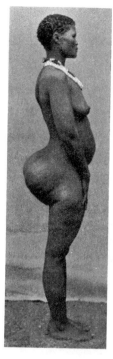

Steatopygia, the prominent fat deposits of the buttocks on this African woman, is a genetic trait, not the product of overeating or sedentary behavior.

jects in the textbooks helped communicate important points about the nature of fattening. I'm going to include some of these photos from seventy or so years ago, so I can make my points more graphically as well. (Modern obesity textbooks, for reasons I've never quite understood, rarely, if ever, include photos of obese humans.) Indeed, much of what we're going to discuss comes straight from these pre–World War II discussions of why we get fat—in particular, from the work of Gustav von Bergmann, the leading German authority on internal medicine in the first half of the twentieth century, and Julius Bauer, a pioneer in the study of hormones and genetics at the University of Vienna, referred to by *The New York Times* in 1930 as the "noted Vienna authority on internal diseases."

It's been known since the 1930s that obesity has a large genetic component. If your parents are fat, it's far more likely you will be fat than someone whose parents are lean. Another way to say this is that body types run in families. Similarities in body types between parents and children and between siblings, as Hilde Bruch said, are often "as striking as facial resemblance." This certainly isn't always the case, just as parents and children don't always look alike. But it's common enough that we all know families in which fathers and sons, mothers and daughters have, in effect, the same bodies. With identical twins, it's not just the faces that look alike; the bodies do as well.

Here are photos of two pairs of identical twins. The first are lean; the second are obese.

In the calories-in/calories-out model, overeating might conceivably tell us why the first pair of twins are slender and the second are not. The pair on the left ate in moderation, balancing

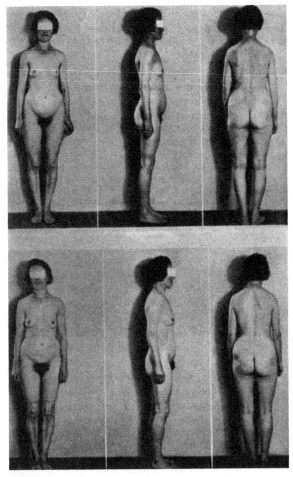

Two pairs of identical twins: one lean, one obese. Did their genes influence how much they ate and exercised or the amount and distribution of their body fat?

calories-in to calories-out with the exquisite accuracy we now know is required; the second pair didn't—they overate. But what about the vertical relationships in the photos? Why do the lean twins have identical bodies? And why do the obese twins? Why is their accumulation of fat so nearly identical? Are we to assume

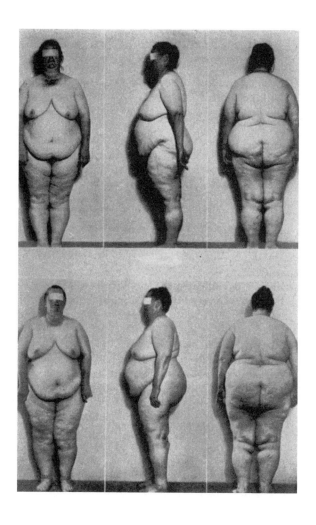

that they just overate, more or less, by exactly the same number of calories over the course of their lives because their genes determined precisely the size of the portions they ate at every meal and precisely how sedentary they chose to be—how many hours they sat on the couch rather than getting up and gardening or walking?

Breeders of livestock have always been implicitly aware of the genetic, constitutional component of fatness. Those engaged in the art and science of animal husbandry have spent many decades breeding cattle, pigs, and sheep to be more fatty or less fatty, just as they breed dairy cattle to increase milk production or dogs for hunting or herding ability. It strains the imagination to believe these livestock breeders are merely manipulating genetic traits that determine the will to eat in moderation and the urge to exercise.

The cow on the top is an Abderdeen Angus, which is bred for the high fat content of its meat. On the bottom is a Jersey cow. It's a lean breed; we can see its ribs protruding through its skin. Jersey cattle are dairy cows, milk producers, which is why the udders on this particular cow are swollen appropriately.

Now, are we to assume, once again, that these Aberdeen Angus cattle are loaded down with what's known in the business as "marbling," or "intramuscular" fat, because they graze longer or more efficiently than the lean Jersey cattle? That the genes of the Aberdeen Angus program them to take bigger bites and so get more calories per hour grazed? Maybe the Jersey cattle get a little more exercise. When the Aberdeen Angus are grazing or sleeping, perhaps the Jersey cattle are loping across the fields, emulating their ancient ancestors who had to run to avoid predators. This sounds absurd, of course, but anything is possible.

The full udders on the Jersey cow and the intramuscular fat on the Aberdeen Angus suggest another possibility. After all, what we want in dairy cattle are animals that convert the maximal amount of energy they consume into milk. This is their utility. We don't want them wasting energy building up fat. With the Aberdeen

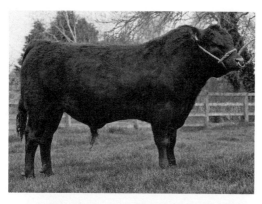

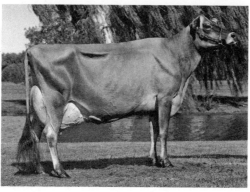

The stocky cow on the top is an Aberdeen Angus; the lean cow on the bottom is a Jersey cow. Their genes probably determine how they partition the calories they consume—into fat, muscle, or milk—not their eating or exercise behavior.

Angus we want an animal that efficiently converts fuel into meat into protein and fat in the muscles. That's where the energy is directed and where it accumulates.

Hence, a likely explanation is that the genes that determine the relative adiposity of these two breeds have little or nothing to do with their appetite or physical activity but, rather, with how they *partition* energy—whether they turn it into protein and fat in the muscles or into milk. The genes don't determine how many calories these animals consume, but what they do with those calories.

Another conspicuous piece of evidence arguing against calories-in/calories-out is that men and women fatten differently. Men typically store fat above the waist—the beer belly—and women below the waist. Women put on fat in puberty, particularly in breasts, hips, butt, and thighs, and men lose fat during puberty and gain muscle.

When boys become men, they become taller, more muscular, and leaner. Girls enter puberty with very slightly more body fat than boys (6 percent more, on average), but by the time puberty is over, they have 50 percent more. "The energy conception can certainly not be applied to this realm," as the German physician Erich Grafe said about this distribution of fat and how it differs by sex in his 1933 textbook *Metabolic Diseases and Their Treatment*. In other words, when a girl enters puberty as slender as a boy and leaves it with the shapely figure of a woman, it's not because of overeating or inactivity, even though it's mostly the fat she's acquired that gives her that womanly shape and she had to eat more calories than she expended to accommodate that fat.

Still more evidence against the conventional wisdom is provided by a very rare disorder known technically as progressive "lipodystrophy." ("Lipo" means "fat"; a "lipodystrophy" is a disorder of fat accumulation.)

By the mid-1950s, some two hundred cases of this disorder had been reported, the great majority in women. It's characterized by the complete loss of subcutaneous fat (the fat immediately beneath the skin) in the upper body, and an excess of fat below the waist. The disorder is called "progressive" because the loss of fat from the upper body progresses with time. It begins with the face and then moves slowly downward to neck, then

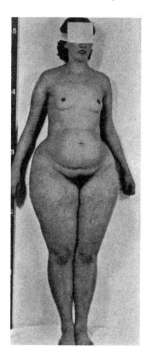

A case of the rare disorder known as "progressive lipodystrophy." At age twenty-four, this woman would be considered obese by today's definition, yet virtually all her body fat was located from her waist down.

shoulders, arms, and trunk. The photo is of a case reported first in 1913.

This young woman began losing the fat from her face when she was ten years old; the fat loss stopped at her waist when she was thirteen. Two years later, she began fattening below the waist. The photo was taken when she was twenty-four; she was five feet four and weighed 185 pounds. By today's standards, she would be considered clinically obese—with a body mass index of almost 32.* But effectively *all* of her body fat was located below her waist. She was as fat as a sumo wrestler from the waist down, as lean as any of the front-runners of an Olympic marathon above it.

So what does this have to do with calories-in/calories-out? If we believe that we get fat because we overeat and we get lean by undereating, are we to assume that these women lost fat on their upper bodies because they underate? And gained fat on their lower bodies because they overate?

This is obviously a ridiculous suggestion. But why is it that when fat loss and fat gain are localized like this—when the obesity or the extreme leanness covers only half the body, or only a

*Body mass index is defined as weight in kilograms divided by the square of height in meters. Obesity is then defined as having a body mass index of 30 or above.

part and not all—they clearly have nothing to do with how much the person ate or exercised; yet when the whole body becomes obese or lean, the difference between calories consumed and expended supposedly explains it?

If this young lady had a few more pounds of fat on her upper body, just enough to soften her features, round out her curves, and if she were to see a doctor today, she would be diagnosed as obese and promptly told to eat less and exercise more. And this would seem perfectly reasonable. But can a valid explanation for obesity and its causes really depend on a few pounds of fat—the difference between sense and nonsense? With these extra pounds, her condition would be blamed on overeating, on the difference between the calories she consumed and expended. Without those extra pounds, with the full lipodystrophy revealed, this explanation becomes nonsensical.

There's a modern example of a lipodystrophy that's not nearly so uncommon—HIV-related lipodystrophy, apparently caused by the anti-retroviral drugs that people infected with HIV take to subdue the virus and keep full-blown AIDS at bay.

These people, too, lose the subcutaneous fat in the face, as

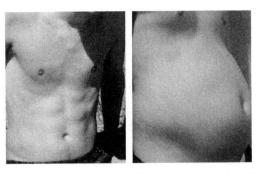

Before and after photos of a man who developed HIV-related lipodystrophy after beginning anti-retroviral therapy.

well as arms, legs, and buttocks, and they also put on fat elsewhere; the gain and loss of fat often happen at different times. They get double chins and a distinctive fat formation on the upper back known as a "buffalo" or "camel hump." Their breasts enlarge, even in men, and they often get a potbelly that looks indistinguishable from the kind we might otherwise attribute to drinking too much beer, as in the case on the previous page. The photo on the left was taken before this patient began antiretroviral therapy for his HIV; the photo on the right was taken four months afterward.

It's hard to imagine, in this case, that eating too much and exercising too little had anything to do with the fat he acquired. And if we can't blame his belly fat on calories-in/calories-out, maybe we shouldn't blame ours, either.

6

Thermodynamics for Dummies, Part 1

The F.D.A. said it wants to initiate a consumer education campaign, focusing on a "calories count" message. After years of promoting a low-fat diet, it is ready to emphasize a new, but actually very old and immutable scientific message: Those who consume more calories than they expend in energy will gain weight. There is no getting around the laws of thermodynamics.

The New York Times, December 1, 2004

There is no getting around the laws of thermodynamics. This certainly is a very old and immutable message. Ever since the early 1900s, when the German diabetes specialist Carl von Noorden first argued that we get fat because we take in more calories than we expend, experts and non-experts alike have insisted that the laws of thermodynamics somehow dictate this to be true.

Arguing to the contrary, that we might actually get fatter for reasons other than the twin sins of overeating and sedentary behavior, or that we might lose fat without consciously eating less and/or exercising more, has invariably been treated as quackery—"emotional and groundless," as the Columbia University physician John Taggart insisted in the 1950s in his introduction to a symposium on obesity. "We have implicit faith in the validity of the first law of thermodynamics." he added.

Such faith is not misplaced. But that does not mean that the laws of thermodynamics have anything more to say about getting fat than any other law of physics. Newton's laws of motion, Einstein's relativity, the electrostatic laws, quantum mechanics—they all describe properties of the universe we no longer question. But they don't tell us why we get fat. They say nothing about it, and this is true of the laws of thermodynamics as well.

It is astounding how much bad science—and so bad advice, and a growing obesity problem—has been the result of the experts' failure to understand this one simple fact. The very notion that we get fat because we consume more calories than we expend would not exist without the misapplied belief that the laws of thermodynamics make it true. When the experts write that "obesity is a disorder of energy balance"—a declaration that can be found in one form or another in much of the technical writing on the subject—it is shorthand for saying that the laws of thermodynamics dictate this to be true. And yet they don't.

Obesity is not a disorder of energy balance or calories-in/calories-out or overeating, and thermodynamics has nothing to do with it. If we can't understand this, we'll keep falling back into the conventional thinking about why we get fat, and that's precisely the trap, the century-old quagmire, that we're trying to avoid.

There are three laws of thermodynamics, but the one that the experts believe is determining why we get fat is the first one. This is also known as the law of energy conservation: all it says is that energy is neither created nor destroyed but can only change from one form to another. Blow up a stick of dynamite, for instance, and the potential energy contained in the chemical bonds of the nitroglycerin is transformed into heat and the kinetic energy of the explosion. Because all mass—our fat tissue, our muscles, our bones, our organs, a planet or star, Oprah Winfrey—is composed of energy, another way to say this is that we can't make something out of nothing or nothing out of something.

Oprah, for instance, can't become more massive—fatter and heavier—without taking in more energy than she expends, because Oprah fatter and heavier contains more energy than Oprah leaner and lighter.* She has to consume more energy than she expends to accommodate her increasing mass. And she can't become leaner and lighter without expending more energy than she takes in. Energy is conserved. That's what this first law of thermodynamics tells us.

This is so simple that the problem with how the experts interpret the law begins to become obvious. All the first law says is that if something gets more or less massive, then more energy or less energy has to enter it than leave it. It says nothing about why this happens. It says nothing about cause and effect. It doesn't tell us why anything happens; it only tells us what has to happen if that thing does happen. A logician would say that it contains no causal information.

Health experts think that the first law is relevant to why we get fat because they say to themselves and then to us, as the *The New York Times* did, "Those who consume more calories than they expend in energy will gain weight." This is true. It has to be. To get fatter and heavier, we *have* to overeat. We have to consume more calories than we expend. That's a given. But thermodynamics tells us nothing about why this happens, *why* we consume more calories than we expend. It only says that if we do, we will get heavier, and if we get heavier, then we did.

Imagine that, instead of talking about why we get fat, we're talking about why a room gets crowded. Now the energy we're discussing is contained in entire people rather than just their fat tissue. Ten people contain so much energy, eleven people contain more, and so on. So what we want to know is why this room is crowded and so overstuffed with energy—that is, people.

If you asked me this question, and I said, *Well, because more*

---

*It is possible to get fatter without getting heavier if we lose muscle and gain fat. Then we don't have to take in more energy than we expend because we might be moving energy from the muscle to the fat. That's why I say fatter and heavier, rather than just fatter.

people entered the room than left it, you'd probably think I was being a wise guy or an idiot. *Of course more people entered than left,* you'd say. *That's obvious. But why?* And, in fact, saying that a room gets crowded because more people are entering than leaving it is redundant—saying the same thing in two different ways—and so meaningless.

Now, borrowing the logic of the conventional wisdom of obesity, I want to clarify this point. So I say, *Listen, those rooms that have more people enter them than leave them will become more crowded. There's no getting around the laws of thermodynamics.* You'd still say, *Yes, but so what?* Or at least I hope you would, because I still haven't given you any causal information. I'm just repeating the obvious.

This is what happens when thermodynamics is used to conclude that overeating makes us fat. Thermodynamics tells us that if we get fatter and heavier, more energy enters our body than leaves it. Overeating means we're consuming more energy than we're expending. It says the same thing in a different way. Neither happens to answer the question why. Why do we take in more energy than we expend? Why do we overeat? Why do we get fatter?*

Answering the "why" question speaks to actual causes. The National Institutes of Health says on its website, "Obesity occurs when a person consumes more calories from food than he or she burns." By using the word "occurs," the NIH experts are not actually saying that overeating is the cause, only a necessary condition. They're being technically correct, but now it's up to us to say,

---

*Jean Mayer, who got a few things right about obesity and weight regulation but the important things wrong, phrased the issue this way back in 1954: "Obesity, too many people believe, is *explained* by overeating; actually it should be recognized that this is simply restating the problem in a different way, and reaffirming (somewhat unnecessarily . . .) one's faith in the First Law of Thermodynamics. To 'explain' obesity by overeating is as illuminating a statement as an 'explanation' of alcoholism by chronic overdrinking."

Okay, so what? Aren't you going to tell us why obesity occurs, rather than tell us what else happens when it does occur?

The experts who say that we get fat *because* we overeat or we get fat *as a result* of overeating—the vast majority—are making the kind of mistake that would (or at least should) earn a failing grade in a high-school science class. They're taking a law of nature that says absolutely nothing about why we get fat and a phenomenon that has to happen if we do get fat—overeating—and assuming these say all that needs to be said. This was a common error in the first half of the twentieth century. It's become ubiquitous since. We need to look elsewhere for answers.

A good place to start might be a National Institutes of Health report published back in 1998. Back then, the NIH experts were a little more forthcoming, and so a little more scientific, about the factors that might cause obesity: "Obesity is a complex, multifactorial chronic disease that develops from an interaction of genotype and the environment," they explained. "Our understanding of how and why obesity develops is incomplete, but involves the integration of social, behavioral, cultural, physiological, metabolic and genetic factors."

So maybe the answers to be found are in this integration of factors—starting with the physiological, metabolic, and genetic ones and letting them lead us to the environmental triggers. Because the one thing we should know for sure is that the laws of thermodynamics, true as they always are, tell us nothing about why we get fat or why we take in more calories than we expend while it's happening.

7

Thermodynamics for Dummies, Part 2

Before leaving thermodynamics behind, let's clear up one more misguided extrapolation of these laws to the world of diet and weight. The very notion that expending more energy than we take in—eating less and exercising more—can cure us of our weight problem, make us permanently leaner and lighter, is based on yet another assumption about the laws of thermodynamics that happens to be incorrect.

The assumption is that the energy we consume and the energy we expend have little influence on each other, that we can consciously change one and it will have no consequence on the other, and vice versa. The thinking is that we can choose to eat less, or semi-starve ourselves (reduce calories-in), and this will have no effect on how much energy we subsequently expend (calories-out) or, for that matter, how hungry we become. We'll feel just as full of pep if we eat twenty-five hundred calories a day as if we consume half that amount. And by the same token, if we increase our expenditure of energy, it will have no influence on how hungry we become (we won't work up an appetite) or on how much energy we expend when we're not exercising.

Intuitively we know this isn't true, and the research in both animals and humans, going back a century, confirms it. People who semi-starve themselves, or who are semi-starved during wars, famines, or scientific experiments, are not only hungry all the time (not to mention cranky and depressed) but lethargic, and they expend less energy. Their body temperatures drop; they tend to be cold all the time. And increasing physical activity *does* increase hunger; exercise does work up an appetite; lumberjacks do eat more than tailors. Physical activity also makes us tired; it wears us out. We expend less energy when the activity is over.

In short, the energy we consume and the energy we expend are dependent on each other. Mathematicians would say they are *dependent* variables, not *independent* variables, as they have typically been treated. Change one, and the other changes to compensate. To a great extent, if not entirely, the energy we expend from day to day and week to week will determine how much we consume, while the energy we consume and make available to our cells (a key point, as I will discuss later) will determine how much we expend. The two are that intimately linked. Anyone who argues differently is treating an extraordinarily complex living organism as though it were a simple mechanical device.

In 2007, Jeffrey Flier, dean of Harvard Medical School and his wife and colleague in obesity research, Terry Maratos-Flier, published an article in *Scientific American* called "What Fuels Fat." In it, they described the intimate link between appetite and energy expenditure, making clear that they are not simply variables that an individual can consciously decide to change with the only effect being that his or her fat tissue will get smaller or larger to compensate.

> An animal whose food is suddenly restricted tends to reduce its energy expenditure both by being less active and by slowing energy use in cells, thereby limiting weight loss. It also experiences increased hunger so that once the restriction ends, it will eat more than its prior norm until the earlier weight is attained.

What the Fliers accomplished in just two sentences is to explain why a hundred years of intuitively obvious dietary advice—eat less—doesn't work in animals. If we restrict the amount of food an animal can eat (we can't just tell it to eat less, we have to give it no choice), not only does it get hungry, but it actually expends less energy. Its metabolic rate slows down. Its cells burn less energy (because they have less energy to burn). And when it gets a chance to eat as much as it wants, it gains the weight right back.

The same is true for humans. I don't know why the Fliers said "an animal" instead of "a person," since the same effects seen in animal studies have been demonstrated repeatedly in humans. One likely answer is that the Fliers (or the magazine's editors) didn't want the implication to be quite so obvious: that the diet advice that our doctors and public-health authorities are invariably giving us is misconceived; that eating less and/or exercising more is not a viable treatment for obesity or overweight and shouldn't be considered as such. It might have short-term effects but nothing that lasts more than a few months or a year. Eventually, our bodies compensate.

8

Head Cases

Of all the dangerous ideas that health officials could have embraced while trying to understand why we get fat, they would have been hard-pressed to find one ultimately more damaging than calories-in/calories-out. That it reinforces what appears to be so obvious—obesity as the penalty for gluttony and sloth—is what makes it so alluring. But it's misleading and misconceived on so many levels that it's hard to imagine how it survived unscathed and virtually unchallenged for the last fifty years.

It has done incalculable harm. Not only is this thinking at least partly responsible for the ever-growing numbers of obese and overweight in the world—while directing attention away from the real reasons we get fat—but it has served to reinforce the perception that those who are fat have no one to blame but themselves. That eating less invariably fails as a cure for obesity is rarely perceived as the single most important reason to make us question our assumptions, as Hilde Bruch suggested half a century ago. Rather, it is taken as still more evidence that the overweight and obese are incapable of following a diet and eating in moderation. And it puts the blame for their physical condition squarely on their behavior, which couldn't be further from the truth.

There has to be a reason, of course, why anyone would eat more calories than he or she expends, particularly since the penalty for doing so is to suffer the physical and emotional cruelties of obesity. There must be a defect involved somewhere; the question is where.

The logic of calories-in/calories-out allows only one acceptable answer to this question. The defect cannot lie in the body—perhaps, as the endocrinologist Edwin Astwood suggested half a century ago, in the "dozens of enzymes" and the "variety of hormones" that control how our bodies "turn what is eaten into fat"—because this would imply that something other than overeating was fundamentally responsible for making us fat. And that's not allowed. So the problem must lie in the brain. And, more precisely, in behavior, which makes it an issue of character. Both eating too much and exercising too little, after all, are behaviors, not physiological states, a fact that's even more obvious if we use the biblical terminology—gluttony and sloth.

The entire science of obesity, in effect, got caught up in the circular logic of the calories-in/calories-out hypothesis, and it's never been able to escape. Establishing the cause of obesity as something that has to happen when people get fat—take in more calories than they expend—prevents any legitimate answer to the question of why anyone would ever do such a thing. Or, at least, why they would do it if they weren't driven to it by forces outside their control.

We have the same problem if we ask why diets fail. Why is it that obesity is so rarely, if ever, cured by what should be the simple act of eating less? If we suggest as an answer that fat people respond to food restriction just as fat animals do—they reduce their energy expenditure, while experiencing increased hunger (as Jeff Flier and Terry Maratos-Flier explained in *Scientific American*)—then we've opened up the possibility that the same physiologic mechanism that drives obese individuals to hold on to their fat in the face of semi-starvation might have been the cause of their obesity in the first place. Again, that's not allowed. So instead we blame the failure of the diet on the failure of the fat person to stay on it. It's a failure of will, a lack of the necessary strength of character to do what lean people do and eat in moderation.

Once overeating is established as the fundamental cause of obesity, blaming behavior—and thus a lack of character and willpower—is the only acceptable explanation. It's the only one that doesn't lend itself to further meaningful research and so, perhaps, the identification of a defect more fundamental still that would explain why people would willingly overeat if they had any choice—that is, why they really got fat.

This insidious logic began to pervade the scientific discussions of obesity in the late 1920s, courtesy of Louis Newburgh, a University of Michigan professor of medicine who would eventually become the most prominent American authority on obesity. Until Newburgh came along, most physicians who thought about obesity assumed that anything so intractable must be a physical disorder, not the end product of a mental state. Newburgh argued the opposite, insisting that those who got fat had a "perverted appetite," which was (for the era) a technical way of saying that these individuals had an urge to consume more calories than they expended, and lean people didn't. Newburgh based this conclusion on the fact that all obese people have literally to overeat to get fatter—which is true, of course, but irrelevant.

This left unanswered, as I said, the obvious questions: Why do people who get fat overeat? Why don't these people control their urges? Why don't they eat in moderation and exercise as lean people do? Well, the choices were no different in Newburgh's era from those we're left with today: fat people are unwilling to make the effort, they lack the willpower, or they're simply unaware of what they should be doing. In short, as Newburgh put it, fat people suffer from "various human weaknesses such as overindulgence and ignorance." (Newburgh himself was lean.)

Had Newburgh's pronouncements been taken with even the slightest bit of skepticism—all medical pronouncements should be, until they are supported by rigorous scientific data—obesity might be far less common today than it is (and this book might not be necessary). But Newburgh was preaching to a medical establishment that had been taught to revere authority figures, not question their pronouncements.

In the United States at least, in the years immediately following the Second World War, Newburgh's word was treated as gospel by a generation of doctors, who should have known better. What they chose to believe is what Newburgh insisted was true, that the obese and overweight belong in one of two categories: those trained since childhood by their parents to take in more food than needed (which was Newburgh's explanation for the observation, clear then as it is now, that a predisposition to obesity runs in families), and those in whom "the combination of weak will and a pleasure seeking outlook upon life" is to blame. And this has been the prevailing attitude ever since, though it is inexcusably simplistic and wrong.

The only thing that's changed over the years is that the experts now couch the concept in ways that don't immediately appear to have such demeaning implications. If we refer to obesity as an eating disorder, for example, as has been common since the 1960s, we're not actually saying that the obese can't eat like the lean because they lack the willpower—we're only saying that they *don't* eat like the lean.

Maybe those who get fat are just too susceptible to external food cues, which was one common explanation in the 1970s, and not susceptible enough to internal cues, which tell them when they've eaten enough but not too much. This doesn't say explicitly that they lack willpower; it suggests instead that something about the brains of obese people makes it harder for them than for lean people to resist the smell of a cinnamon bun or the sight of a McDonald's. Or they're more likely to order a larger portion or keep eating it, whereas a lean person either wouldn't order it to begin with or wouldn't feel compelled to finish it.*

---

*Julius Bauer, a University of Vienna professor, had a much more rational way of thinking about obesity, which I will discuss shortly. "Those who still

By the 1970s, an entire field of what's technically (and tellingly) called "behavioral medicine" had emerged to treat obese individuals with behavioral therapies, all subtle or not so subtle ways of inducing the obese to behave like the lean, that is, to eat in moderation.[†] None of these therapies has ever been shown to work; many are still us with us today even so. Slowing down the pace of eating is a typical behavioral treatment. Not eating anywhere other than in the kitchen or at the dining-room table is another one.

Today it's still the case that many, if not most, of the leading authorities on obesity are psychologists and psychiatrists, people whose expertise is meant to be in the ways of the mind, not of the body. Imagine how many more dead diabetics we'd have if victims of that disease were treated by psychologists instead of physicians. And yet diabetes and obesity are so closely linked—most type 2 diabetics are obese, and many obese people become diabetic—that some authorities have taken to calling the two disorders "diabesity," as though they're two sides of the same pathological coin, which they assuredly are.

Much of the last half-century of professional discourse on obesity can be perceived as attempts to circumvent what we could call the "head case" implications of calories-in/calories-out: how to blame obesity on eating too much without actually blaming the fat person for the human weaknesses of self-indulgence and/or

---

believe that the problem of obesity is exhausted by the statement that there is an imbalance between intake and output of energy," he wrote prophetically in 1947, "assume that only a particular behavior—the craving for food on the basis of emotional reasons—accounts for overeating and subsequent obesity. Do these authors wish to range obesity as a 'behavioral problem' among psychiatric instead of metabolic diseases? This would be at least the logical though absurd consequence of their theory."

[†]Moderation, of course, would have to be defined as little enough so that weight would actually be lost, an amount that could be significantly smaller than that consumed by a lean person of similar height and bone structure.

ignorance. If the obesity epidemic is blamed on "prosperity," as I discussed earlier, or a "toxic food environment," we can shift the responsibility for obesity away from the character of the obese while still recognizing that they only got that way by failing to eat in moderation. If the food industry is blamed for making too much tasty and tempting food available, this further shifts the blame. It's the environment we live in that makes us fat, we're being told, not just our weakness of will. Then why don't lean people get fat in this toxic environment? Is the answer only willpower?

In the 1930s, Russell Wilder of the Mayo Clinic asked the pertinent question of Newburgh's perverted-appetite idea, and that question is still the one we should be asking today when anyone tries to blame society or the food industry for why we get fat: "There must be some device other than appetite to regulate weight because we continue to be protected against obesity, most of us," Wilder said, "even though we hoodwink our appetite by various tricks, such as cocktails and wines with our meals. The whole artistry of cookery, in fact, is developed with the prime object of inducing us to eat more than we ought. Why, then, do we not all grow fat?" If some of us don't, why not? Why are some of us protected from obesity despite the "whole artistry of cookery" and some not?

In 1978, Susan Sontag published an essay called *Illness as Metaphor*, in which she discussed cancer and tuberculosis and the "blame the victim" mentality that often accompanied these diseases in different eras. "Theories that diseases are caused by mental states and can be cured by will power," Sontag wrote, "are always an index of how much is not understood about the physical terrain of a disease."

So long as we believe that people get fat because they overeat, because they take in more calories than they expend, we're putting the ultimate blame on a mental state, a weakness of character, and we're leaving human biology out of the equation entirely. Sontag had it right: it's a mistake to think this way about any disease. And it's been disastrous when it comes to the question of why we get fat. How *should* we be approaching the problem? How do we have to think about it to make progress? Those are the questions I'll begin to answer in the next chapter.

BOOK II

Adiposity 101

9

The Laws of Adiposity

The fate of the laboratory rat is rarely enviable. The story I'm about to tell offers no exception. Still, we can learn from the rat's experience, as scientists do.

In the early 1970s, a young researcher at the University of Massachusetts named George Wade set out to study the relationship between sex hormones, weight, and appetite by removing the ovaries from rats (females, obviously) and then monitoring their subsequent weight and behavior.* The effects of the surgery were suitably dramatic: the rats would begin to eat voraciously and quickly become obese. If we didn't know any better, we might assume from this that the removal of a rat's ovaries makes it a glutton. The rat eats too much, the excess calories find their way to the fat tissue, and the animal becomes obese. This would confirm our preconception that overeating is responsible for obesity in humans as well.

But Wade did a revealing second experiment, removing the ovaries from the rats and putting them on a strict postsurgical diet. Even if these rats were ravenously hungry after the surgery, even if they desperately wanted to be gluttons, they couldn't satisfy their urge. In the lingo of experimental science, this second experi-

---

*The tendency in popular science and medical writing is to make it appear that one researcher did all the work, so as not to clutter up the prose by having to keep repeating phrases like "Wade and his students." I'm doing the same here. Wade did these experiments with various undergraduates and graduate students. The work was collaborative, as science almost always is.

ment *controlled* for overeating. The rats, postsurgery, were only allowed the same amount of food they would have eaten had they never had the surgery.

What happened is not what you'd probably think. The rats got just as fat, just as quickly. But these rats were now completely sedentary. They moved only when movement was required to get food.

If we knew only about the second experiment, this, too, might confirm our preconceptions. Now we would assume that removing a rat's ovaries makes it lazy; it expends too little energy, and this is why it gets fat. In this interpretation, once again we have support for our belief in the primacy of calories-in/calories-out as the determining factor in obesity.

Pay attention to both experiments, though, and the conclusion is radically different. Removing the ovaries from a rat literally makes its fat tissue absorb calories from the circulation and expand with fat. If the animal can eat more to compensate for the calories that are now being stashed away as fat (the first experiment), it will. If it can't (the second), then it expends less energy, because it now has fewer calories available to expend.

The way Wade explained it to me, the animal doesn't get fat because it overeats, it overeats because it's getting fat. The cause and effect are reversed. Both gluttony and sloth are effects of the drive to get fatter. They are caused fundamentally by a defect in the regulation of the animal's fat tissue. The removal of the ovaries literally makes the rat stockpile body fat; the animal either eats more or expends less energy, or both, to compensate.

To explain why this happens, I'm going to have to get technical for a moment. As it turns out, removing the rats' ovaries serves the function of removing estrogen, the female sex hormone that is normally secreted by the ovaries. (When estrogen was infused back into the rats postsurgery, they did not eat voraciously, become slothful, or grow obese. They acted like perfectly normal rats.) And one of the things that estrogen does in rats (and humans) is influence an enzyme called lipoprotein lipase—LPL,

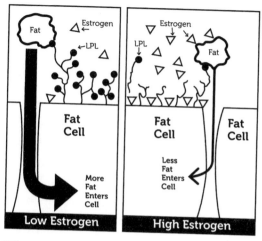

When estrogen levels are low (left), the enzyme LPL is "upregulated" on fat cells, and more fat is pulled from the circulation into the cell. When estrogen levels are high (right), LPL activity is suppressed, and the fat cells accumulate less fat.

for short. What LPL does in turn, very simplistically, is to pull fat from the bloodstream into whatever cell happens to "express" this LPL. If the LPL is attached to a fat cell, then it pulls fat from the circulation into the fat cell. The animal (or the person) in which that fat cell resides gets infinitesimally fatter. If the LPL is attached to a a muscle cell, it pulls the fat into the muscle cell, and the muscle cell burns it for fuel.*

Estrogen happens to suppress or "inhibit" the activity of LPL on fat cells. The more estrogen around, the less LPL will be pulling fat out of the bloodstream and into the fat cells, and the less fat those cells will accumulate. Get rid of the estrogen (by removing the ovaries) and fat cells blossom with LPL. The LPL

---

*This is how *Williams Textbook of Endocrinology*, a well-respected textbook on hormones and hormone-related diseases, describes this same concept: "The activity of LPL within individual tissues is a key factor in partitioning triglycerides [i.e., fat] among different body tissues."

then does what it always does—pull fat into the cells—but now the animal gets far fatter than normal, because now the fat cells have far more LPL doing that job.

The animal has the urge to eat voraciously because it's now losing calories into its fat cells that are needed elsewhere to run its body. The more calories its fat cells sequester, the more it must eat to compensate. The fat cells, in effect, are hogging calories, and there aren't enough to go around for other cells. Now a meal that would previously have satisfied the animal no longer does. And because the animal is getting fatter (and heavier), this increases its caloric requirements even further. So the animal is ravenous, and if it can't satisfy its newfound hunger, it has to settle for expending less energy.

The only way (short of more surgery) to stop these animals from getting fat—dieting has no effect, and we can be confident that trying to force them to exercise would be futile—is to give them their estrogen back. When that is done, they become lean again, and their appetite and energy levels return to normal.

So removing the ovaries from a rat literally makes its fat cells fatten. And this, very likely, is what happens to many women who get fat when they have their ovaries removed or after menopause. They secrete less estrogen, and their fat cells express more LPL.

The story of these ovariectomized rats reverses our perception of the cause and effect of obesity. It tells us that two behaviors—gluttony and sloth—that seem to be the reasons we get fat can in fact be the effects of getting fat. It tells us that if we pay attention to the hormones and enzymes that regulate the fat tissue itself, we can understand precisely why this is so: not only why these rats get fat but why they exhibit the behaviors that we typically associate with fat people.

Another remarkable aspect of the last half-century of discussion about obesity and weight loss is that medical experts have been remarkably uninterested in the fat tissue itself and how our bodies happen to regulate it. With very few exceptions, they've simply ignored the fat tissue because they've already concluded that the problem is behavioral and lies in the brain, not in the body. Had we been discussing disorders of growth—why some people grow to be more than seven feet tall and others never make it to four feet—the only subject of discussion would be the hormones and enzymes that regulate growth. And yet, when we're discussing a disorder in which the defining symptom is the abnormal growth of our fat tissue, the hormones and enzymes that regulate that growth are considered irrelevant.*

When we pay attention to the regulation of our fat tissue, though, we arrive at an explanation for why we get fat and what to do about it that differs radically from the conventional thinking derived from the focus on the balance of energy consumed and expended. We have to conclude, as Wade did for his rats, that those who get fat do so because of the way their fat happens to be regulated and that a conspicuous consequence of this regulation is to cause the eating behavior (gluttony) and the physical inactivity (sloth) that we so readily assume are the actual causes.

I'm going to discuss this idea first as a hypothesis, a way of thinking about why we get fat that could be correct, and then I'm going to explain why it almost assuredly is.† Before I get to that, though, there are several critical points about fat and the process

---

*The Wikipedia entry for "obesity" in July 2009, when I wrote this chapter, included no discussion of the regulation of fat issue, although that could be found in the entry for "adipose tissue." The implicit assumption would be that the regulation of fat tissue is not relevant to a disorder of excess fat accumulation.

†When I use the phrase "almost assuredly," what I mean is that I believe this to be the case with such conviction that I would stake my reputation on it. But I've been writing about science so long, and am such a firm believer in the process of science, that I find I can't remove the "almost." We can never say anything for certain in science until it has survived rigorous tests, particularly when we're challenging accepted beliefs. When people do, it's a good reason not to trust them, whether they are diet-book authors or academic experts. Nonetheless, if you prefer to read "almost assuredly" as "assuredly," you'll almost assuredly be justified in doing so.

of fattening itself that you'll have to understand. In honor of the laws of thermodynamics that they're replacing, we'll call these the laws of adiposity.

The First Law

Body fat is carefully regulated, if not exquisitely so.

This is true even though some people fatten so easily that it's virtually impossible to imagine. What I mean by "regulated" is that our bodies, when healthy, are working diligently to maintain a set amount of fat in our fat tissue—not too much and not too little—and that this, in turn, is used to assure a steady supply of fuel to the cells. The implication (our working assumption) is that if someone gets obese it's because this regulation has been thrown out of whack, not that it's ceased to exist.

The evidence that fat tissue is carefully regulated, not just a garbage can where we dump whatever calories we don't burn, is incontrovertible. We can start with all the observations in chapter 5 about the wheres, whens, and whos of fattening. That men and women fatten differently tells us that sex hormones play a role in regulating body fat (as do Wade's experiments and what we know about estrogen and LPL). That some parts of our bodies are relatively fat free—the backs of our hands, for example, and our foreheads—and others not so, tells us that local factors play a role in where we fatten. Just as local factors obviously play a role in where we grow hair—in some places, but not in others.

That obesity runs in families (we're more likely to be fat if our parents were fat) and that the local distribution of fat itself can be a genetic attribute (the steatopygia of certain African tribes) tells us that body fat is regulated, because how else would the genes passed from generation to generation influence our fat and where we put it, if not through the hormones and enzymes and other factors that regulate it?

That the amount of fat (and even the type of fat) animals carry is carefully regulated also argues for this conclusion. We are, after all, just another species of animal. Animals in the wild may be naturally fat (hippopotami, for instance, and whales). They'll put on fat seasonally, as insulation in preparation for the cold of winter or as fuel for annual migrations or hibernations. Females will fatten in preparation for giving birth; males will fatten to give them a weight advantage in fights for females. But they *never* get obese, meaning they won't suffer adverse health consequences from their fat the way humans do. They won't become diabetic, for instance.

No matter how abundant their food supply, wild animals will maintain a stable weight—not too fat, not too thin—which tells us that their bodies are assuring that the amount of fat in their fat tissue always works to their advantage and never becomes a hindrance to survival. When animals do put on significant fat, that fat is always there for a very good reason.* The animals will be as healthy with it as without.

Excellent examples of how carefully animals (and so presumably humans, too) regulate their fat accumulation are hibernating rodents—ground squirrels, for example, which double their weight and body fat in just a few weeks of late summer. Dissecting these squirrels at their peak weight, as one researcher described it to me, is like "opening a can of Crisco oil—enormous gobs of fat, all over the place."

But these squirrels will accumulate this fat regardless of how much they eat, just like Wade's ovary-less rats. They can be housed in a laboratory and kept to a strict diet from springtime, when they awake from hibernation, through late summer, and they'll get just as fat as squirrels allowed to eat to their hearts' content. They'll

---

*The camel's hump is another example of a large fat mass that exists for a purpose: the hump provides a reservoir of fat for survival in the desert, without the camel's having to keep that fat in subcutaneous deposits, as we do, where the insulation would present problems in the desert heat. The same goes for fat-rumped and fat-tailed sheep, and fat-tailed marsupial mice, all desert dwellers that carry their fat almost exclusively in the eponymous locations.

burn the fat through the winter and lose it at the same rate, whether they remain awake in a warm laboratory with food available or go into full hibernation, eating not a bite, and surviving solely off their fat supplies.

The fact is, there's very little that researchers can do to keep these animals from gaining and losing fat on schedule. Manipulating the food available, short of virtually starving them to death, is not effective. The amount of fat on these rodents at any particular time of the year is regulated entirely by biological factors, not by the food supply itself or the amount of energy required to get that food. And this makes perfect sense. If an animal that requires enormous gobs of fat for its winter fuel were to require excessive amounts of food to accumulate that fat, then one bad summer would have long ago wiped out the entire species.

It may be true that evolution has singled out humans as the sole species on the planet whose bodies do not work to regulate fat stores carefully in response to periods of both feast and famine, that some people will stockpile so much fat merely because food is available in abundance that they become virtually immobile, but accepting this conclusion requires that we ignore virtually everything we know about evolution.

A final argument for the careful regulation of body fat is the fact that everything else in our bodies is meticulously regulated. Why would fat be an exception? When regulation breaks down, as it does in cancer and heart disease, the result is often fatally obvious. When people accumulate excess fat, this tells us that something has gone awry in the careful regulation of their fat tissue. What we need to know is what that defect is and what to do about it.

The Second Law

Obesity can be caused by a regulatory defect so small that it would be undetectable by any technique yet invented.

Remember the twenty-calorie-a-day problem I discussed earlier? If we overeat by just twenty calories each day—adding just 1 percent or less to our typical daily caloric quota, without a compensatory increase in expenditure—that's enough to transform us from lean in our twenties to obese in our fifties. In the context of the calories-in/calories-out logic, this led to the obvious question: How do any of us remain lean if it requires that we consciously balance the calories we eat to those we expend with an accuracy of better than 1 percent? That seems impossible, and assuredly is.

Well, these same twenty calories a day is all this regulatory system has to misdirect into our fat cells to make us obese. The same arithmetic applies. If, by some unlucky combination of genes and environment, a regulatory error causes our fat cells to store an excess of just 1 percent of the calories that would otherwise be used for fuel, then we are destined to become obese.

If this misappropriation of calories into fat is only slightly larger, someone could end up grotesquely fat. Yet this would still seem like a relatively minor error in regulatory judgment—just a few percentage points, something exceedingly difficult to measure and yet not that hard to imagine.

The Third Law

Whatever makes us both fatter and heavier will also make us overeat.

This was the ultimate lesson of Wade's rats. It may be counterintuitive, but it *has* to be true for every species, for every person who puts on pounds of fat. It's arguably the one lesson we (and our health experts) have to learn in order to understand why we get fat and what to do about it.

This law is one fact we can count on from the first law of thermodynamics, the law of energy conservation, which health experts have been so determined to misapply. *Anything* that increases its mass, for whatever reason, will take in more energy than it expends. So, if a regulatory defect makes us both fatter and heavier, it is guaranteed to make us consume more calories (and so increase our appetite) and/or expend less than would be the case if this regulation was working perfectly.

Here's where growing children help as a metaphor to understand this cause and effect of getting fat and overeating. I'm going to use two photos of my oldest son to make this point. The photo below, on the left, was taken when he was not quite two years old and weighed thirty-four pounds.

The photo on the right was taken three years later, after he had gained nine inches in height and weighed fifty-one pounds.

He gained seventeen pounds in three years, so he certainly consumed more calories than he expended. He overate. Those excess calories were used to create all the necessary tissues and structures that a larger body needed, including, yes, even more fat. But he didn't grow because he consumed excess calories. He consumed those excess calories—he overate—because he was growing.

My son's growth, like every child's, is caused fundamentally by the action of growth hormones. As he gets older, he'll occasionally go through growth spurts that will be accompanied by a

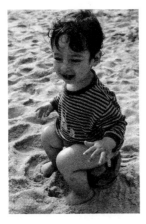 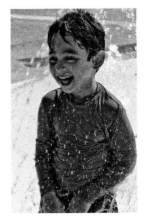

August 2007—thirty-four pounds   *August 2010—fifty-one pounds*

98

voracious appetite and probably a fair share of sloth, but the appetite and the sloth will be driven by the growth, not vice versa. His body will require excess calories to satisfy the demands of the growth—to build a bigger body—and it will figure out a way to get them, by increasing his appetite or decreasing his energy expenditure or both. When he goes through puberty, he'll lose fat and gain muscle; he'll still be taking in more calories than he expends, and this, too, will be driven by hormonal changes.

That growth is the cause and overeating the effect is almost assuredly true for our fat tissue as well. To paraphrase what the German internist Gustav von Bergmann said about this idea more than eighty years ago, we would never even consider the possibility that children grow taller because they eat too much and exercise too little (or that they stunt their growth by exercising too much). So why assume that these are valid explanations for growing fat (or remaining lean)? "That which the body needs to grow it always finds," von Bergmann wrote, "and that which it needs to become fat, even if it's ten times as much, the body will save for itself from the annual balance."

The only reason to think that this isn't true, that the cause and effect go in one direction when we get taller (growth causes overeating) and the other when we grow fatter (overeating causes growth), is that this is what we grew up believing and we never stopped to consider if it actually makes sense. The far more reasonable assumption is that growth in both cases determines appetite and even energy expenditure—not the other way around. We don't get fat because we overeat; we overeat because we're getting fat.

Since this is so counterintuitive but so critical to understand, I want to return to the examples of animals. African elephants are the world's largest land animals. The males typically weigh more than ten thousand pounds, although surprisingly little of this is fat. Blue whales are the largest animals, on or off land. They can weigh three hundred thousand pounds, and much of that is fat. African elephants will eat hundreds of pounds of food a day, and blue whales, thousands,* prodigious amounts, but neither species grow to be enormous because they eat so much. They eat prodigious amounts because they're enormous animals. With or without large quantities of body fat, body size determines how much they eat.

The infants of these species also eat relatively enormous quantities. They do so because they're born exceedingly large to begin with and because their genes predispose them to grow many thousands of pounds (elephants) or hundreds of thousands of pounds (blue whales) larger still. Now both growth *and* body size are driving appetite. This is true whether these animals are using the calories to store fat, or to enlarge muscle and other tissues and organs. Whether or not they have enormous quantities of fat, the same cause and effect holds true.

Now consider what researchers call animal models of obesity—animals, like Wade's rats, that are made obese in the laboratory but wouldn't be naturally. Over the past eighty years, researchers have learned that they can make rats and mice obese by breeding, by surgery (removing the ovaries, for instance), by the manipulation of their diets, and by any number of genetic manipulations. The animals on which these indignities are inflicted do indeed become obese, not just functionally fat (like blue whales or hibernating ground squirrels). They tend to suffer from the same metabolic disturbances, including diabetes, that we do when we become obese.

It doesn't matter, though, what technique is used to make the animals obese; they'll still get that way, or at least significantly fatter (just as Wade's rats did), whether or not they can eat any more calories than otherwise identical animals that remain lean. They

---

*This is only in summer. During the rest of the year, whales apparently live off their stored fat, like hibernating rodents.

get obese not because they overeat but because the surgery or breeding or genetic manipulation or even the change in diet has disturbed the regulation of their fat tissue. They begin stockpiling calories as fat, and then their bodies have to compensate: they eat more, if possible; they expend less energy if not. Often they do both.*

Take, for example, the preferred method of making laboratory rodents obese from the 1930s through the 1960s. This was a surgical technique that required inserting a needle into a part of the brain known as the hypothalamus, which controls (not coincidentally) hormone secretion throughout the body. After the surgery, some of these rodents would eat voraciously and get obese; some would become sedentary and get obese; some would do both and get obese. The obvious conclusion, suggested first by the neuroanatomist Stephen Ranson, whose Northwestern University laboratory pioneered these experiments in the 1930s, is that the surgery has the direct effect of increasing body fat on these rodents. After the surgery, their fat tissue sucks up calories to make more fat; this leaves insufficient fuel for the rest of the body—what Ranson called "hidden semi-cellular starvation"—and "force[s] the body either to increase its general food intake or to cut down its expenditure, or both."

The only way to prevent these animals from getting obese is to starve them—to inflict what a Johns Hopkins University physiologist in the 1940s called "severe and permanent" food restriction. If these animals are allowed to eat even moderate amounts of food, they end up obese. In other words, they get fat not by *overeating* but by eating at all. Even though the surgery is in the brain, it has

---

*To be more precise, every animal model of obesity that researchers study in the laboratory (to the best of my knowledge) can be divided into two categories: (1) those in which this same cause and effect holds true, and (2) those in which the researchers never thought to do the experiments to find out (put the animals on a calorie-restricted diet and see if they get fat anyway), because the researchers never imagined that their animals might get fat for any reason other than eating too much.

the effect of fundamentally altering the regulation of body fat, not appetite.

The same thing holds true for animals that are bred to be obese, for which obesity is in their genes. In the 1950s, Jean Mayer studied one such strain of obese mice in his Harvard laboratory. As he reported it, he could get their *weight* below that of lean mice if he starved them sufficiently, but they'd "still contain more fat than the normal ones, while their muscles have melted away." Once again, eating too much wasn't the problem; these mice, as Mayer wrote, "will make fat out of their food under the most unlikely circumstances, even when half starved."

Then there are Zucker rats. Researchers began studying these rats in the 1960s, and they are still a favorite obesity model today. Here's a picture of a Zucker rat looking suitably corpulent.

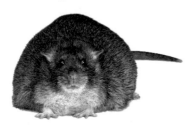

These rats, like Mayer's mice, are genetically predisposed to get fat. When Zucker rats are put on a calorie-restricted diet from the moment they're weaned from their mothers' milk, they don't end up leaner than their litter-mates who are allowed to eat as much as they want. They end up fatter. They may weigh a little less, but they have just as much or even more body fat. Even if they want to be gluttons, which they assuredly do, they can't, and they still get even fatter than they would have had they never been put on a diet. On the other hand, their muscles and organs, including their brains and kidneys, are smaller than they'd otherwise be. Just as the muscles in Mayer's mice "melted away" when starved, the muscles and organs in these semi-starved Zucker rats are "significantly reduced" in size compared with those fat littermates who get to eat freely. "In order to develop this obese body composition in the face of calorie restriction," wrote the researcher who reported this observation in 1981, "several developing organ systems in the obese rats [are] compromised."

The Laws of Adiposity

Let's think about this for a second. If a baby rat that is genetically programmed to become obese is put on a diet from the moment it's weaned, so it can eat no more than a lean rat would eat, if that, and can *never* eat as much as it would like, it responds by *compromising* its organs and muscles to satisfy its genetic drive to grow fat. It's not just using the energy it would normally expend in day-to-day activity to grow fat; it's taking the materials and the energy it would normally dedicate to building its muscles, organs, and even its brain and using that.

When these obese rodents are starved to death—an experiment that fortunately not too many researchers have done—a common result reported in the literature is that the animals die with much of their fat tissue intact. In fact, they'll often die with more body fat than lean animals have when the lean ones are eating as much as they like. As animals starve, and the same is true of humans, they consume their muscles for fuel, and that includes, eventually, the heart muscle. As adults, these obese animals are willing to compromise their organs, even their hearts and their lives, to preserve their fat.

The message of eighty years of research on obese animals is simple and unconditional and worth restating: obesity does not come about because gluttony and sloth make it so; only a change in the regulation of the fat tissue makes a lean animal obese.

The amount of body fat on obese animals is determined by a balance of all the various forces that work on the fat tissue—on the fat cells, as we'll see—either to put fat in or to get fat out. Whatever has been done to these animals to make them fat (surgery, genetic manipulation), the effect is literally to change this balance of forces so that the animals increase their fat stores. Now "eating too much" is a meaningless concept, because otherwise normal amounts of food are now "too much." The fat tissue is not reacting to how much these animals are eating but only to the forces making them accumulate fat. And because increasing body fat requires energy and nutrients that are needed elsewhere in their bodies, they will eat more if they can. If they can't—if they are on a strict diet—they will expend less energy, because they have less to expend. They may even compromise their brains, muscles, and other organs. Half-starve these animals and they'll still find a way to stockpile calories as fat, because that's what their fat tissue is now programmed to do.

If this is true of humans, and there's little reason to think it's not, it is the explanation for the paradigm-challenging observation I mentioned earlier, regarding extremely poor but overweight mothers with thin, stunted children. Both mother and children are, indeed, half-starved. The emaciated children, their growth stunted, respond as we'd expect. The mothers, however, have fat tissue that has developed its own agenda (we'll see shortly how this can happen). It will accumulate excess fat, and does so, even though the mothers themselves, like their children, are barely getting enough food to survive. They must be expending less energy to compensate.

Before I leave the laws of adiposity and this animal research behind, I want to ask one more question: What do these laws and this research have to say about people who are habitually lean? Over the years, researchers have also created what we might call animal models of leanness—animals whose genes have been manipulated so they are leaner than they'd otherwise be. These animals will remain lean even when the researchers force them to consume more calories than they prefer—by infusing nutrients through a tube into their guts, for instance, pumping in calories directly. In such cases, the animals will surely have to increase their expenditure to burn off the calories.*

The implication is as counterintuitive as anything we've discussed so far. Just as the animal research tells us that gluttony and sloth are side effects of a drive to accumulate body fat, it also says that eating in moderation and being physically active (literally, having the energy to exercise) are not evidence of moral recti-

---

*These researchers typically don't measure energy expenditure in these rodents, so I'm assuming this is true.

tude. Rather, they're the metabolic benefits of a body that's programmed to remain lean. If our fat tissue is regulated so that it will *not* store significant calories as fat, or our muscle tissue is regulated to take up more than its fair share of calories to use for fuel, then we'll either eat less than those of us predisposed to be fat (the first case), or we'll be more physically active (the second), or both, because of it.

This implies that our emaciated marathoners are not lean because they train religiously and burn off thousands of calories doing so; rather, they're driven to expend those calories—and so perhaps to work out for hours a day and become obsessive long-distance runners—because they're wired to burn off calories and be lean. Similarly, a greyhound will be more physically active than a basset hound, not because of any conscious desire to exercise, but because its body partitions fuel to its lean tissue, not to its fat.

It may be easier to believe that we remain lean because we're virtuous and we get fat because we're not, but the evidence simply says otherwise. Virtue has little more to do with our weight than with our height. When we grow taller, it's hormones and enzymes that are promoting our growth, and we consume more calories than we expend as a result. Growth is the cause—increased appetite and decreased energy expenditure (gluttony and sloth) are the effects. When we grow fatter, the same is true as well.

We don't get fat because we overeat; we overeat because we're getting fat.

10

A Historical Digression on "Lipophilia"

This way of thinking about why we get fat is by no means original, as I've suggested. It dates to 1908, when the German internist Gustav von Bergmann evoked the term "lipophilia"—"love of fat"—to explain why parts of the body differ in their affinity for stockpiling fat. (One of the highest honors awarded today by the German Society of Internal Medicine is in honor of von Bergmann.) In essence, I'm doing little more in this book than taking von Bergmann's ideas and updating the science.

Von Bergmann's approach to obesity was straightforward: he considered it a disorder of excess fat accumulation and then set out to learn what he could about the regulation of our fat tissue. His observations—many of which I cited earlier—led him to the conclusion that some tissue is obviously "lipophilic" and avidly accumulates fat, and other tissue is not. This attribute, he noted, differs not only from tissue to tissue but from person to person. Just as some parts of the body have an affinity for growing hair and others don't, and some people are hairier than others, some have an affinity for accumulating fat and others don't, and some people are fatter (their bodies are more lipophilic) than others. These people fatten easily, and it often seems there's nothing they can do about it. Others, whose bodies are not lipophilic, are lean; they find it difficult to put on weight, even if they make a concerted effort.

A Historical Digression on "Lipophilia"

In the late 1920s, von Bergmann's lipophilia idea was taken up and championed by Julius Bauer of the University of Vienna. Bauer was a pioneer in the application of genetics and endocrinology to clinical medicine, at a time when these sciences were in their infancy.* Few physicians of that era could imagine how genes might bestow lifelong characteristics on people and, with them, a predisposition for disease. Bauer knew more about this relationship between genes and disease than anyone, and he spent considerable effort trying to get physicians in the United States to see the errors in Louis Newburgh's "perverted appetite" hypothesis.

Whereas Newburgh argued that genes, if they did anything (which he doubted), *might* bestow on the obese an uncontrollable urge to eat too much, Bauer explained that the only way genes could logically cause obesity is by directly influencing the regulation of the fat tissue itself. They "regulate lipophilia," he said, and then this regulation, in turn, determines "the general feelings ruling the intake of food and the expenditure of energy."

Bauer considered the fat tissue in obesity akin to malignant tumors. Both have their own agendas, he explained. Tumors are driven to grow and spread and will do so with little relation to how much the person who has that tumor might be eating or exercising. In those who are predisposed to grow obese, fat tissue is driven to grow, to expand with fat, and it will accomplish this goal, just as the tumor does, with little concern about what the rest of the body might be doing. "The abnormal lipophilic tissue seizes on foodstuffs, even in the case of undernutrition," Bauer wrote in 1929. "It maintains its stock, and may increase it independent of the requirements of the organism. A sort of anarchy exists; the adipose tissue lives for itself and does not fit into the precisely regulated management of the whole organism."

*"His lectures (held in English) were much sought after by physicians from the United Kingdom and the United States," *The Lancet* wrote when Bauer died in 1979, at the age of ninety-two.

By the late 1930s, von Bergmann and Bauer's lipophilia hypothesis had become "more or less fully accepted" in Europe.* It was catching on in the United States as well, where Russell Wilder of the Mayo Clinic wrote in 1938, "This conception deserves attentive consideration."

Within a decade, though, it had vanished. Those European physicians and researchers who hadn't died in the Second World War or fled the continent (as Bauer did in 1938) had far more pressing issues to deal with than obesity. In the United States, a new generation of physicians and nutritionists came along after the war to fill the void, and they were enamored with Newburgh's "perverted appetite" logic, perhaps because it played to their preconceptions about the penalties of gluttony and sloth.

Anti-German sentiment in the postwar medical community, understandable as it may have been, assuredly didn't help matters. The authorities writing about obesity in the United States after the war treated the German medical literature as though it didn't exist, even though it was Germans and Austrians who had founded and done most of the meaningful research in the fields of nutrition, metabolism, endocrinology, and genetics, which means all the fields relevant to obesity. (The one notable exception was Hilde Bruch, a German herself, who discussed this prewar literature extensively.) Once the psychologists took over in the 1960s and obesity officially became an eating disorder—a character defect but in kinder words—any hope that these authorities would pay attention to how the fat tissue was regulated effectively vanished.

Still, a few research-oriented physicians occasionally came to the same conclusions after the war. Bruch, who remained the leading authority on childhood obesity through the 1960s, continued to suggest that a defect in the regulation of fat tissue was the

---

*The quote is from *Obesity and Leanness*, a textbook by the Northwestern University Medical School endocrinologist Hugo Rony, which was published in 1940.

likely cause of obesity and professed amazement that her colleagues were so completely uninterested in the idea. Even Jean Mayer, as late as 1968, was pointing out that "different body types and fat contents" were associated with "different concentrations of hormones in the blood" and suggesting that slight differences in "relative or absolute hormone concentrations" might be the reason why some get fat and others stay effortlessly lean. In other words, as von Bergmann and Bauer would have said, these hormone concentrations might be determining whether or not fat tissue is lipophilic. (Mayer paid no attention to what von Bergmann and Bauer had written, or neglected to credit them if he did.)

The postwar expert who had the most perceptive take on why we get fat happened to be the one who had the most expertise in hormones and hormone-related disorders—Edwin Astwood of Tufts University. In 1962, Astwood was president of the Endocrinology Society when he gave a lecture called "The Heritage of Corpulence" at its annual meeting. Astwood attacked the notion that obesity was caused by overeating—"the primacy of gluttony," as he described this way of thinking—and his presentation was as good a description as any I know on the subject of how we can think about obesity if we simply focus on the fat and the fat tissue, attend to the actual evidence (always a good idea), and do so with no preconceptions (also a good idea).

The first point that Astwood made was that a predisposition to fatten easily or remain lean is obviously determined in large part by our genes—a heritage, something passed down from generation to generation. If genes determine our height and our hair color and the size of our feet, he said, then "why can't heredity be credited with determining one's shape?"

But if genes control our shape, how do they do it? By 1962, biochemists and physiologists had gone a long way toward establishing exactly how body fat is regulated, as I will discuss shortly, and Astwood considered this to be the obvious answer, just as von Bergmann, Bauer, and Bruch had before him. Dozens of enzymes and multiple hormones had already been identified that influence fat accumulation, Astwood explained. Some work to liberate fat from the fat tissue; others to put it there. Ultimately, the amount of fat that would be stored in any single person or at any single location on the human body would be determined by the balance of these competing regulatory forces.

"Now just suppose that any one of these . . . regulatory processes were to go awry," Astwood said.

Suppose that the release of fat or its combustion [burning it for fuel] was somewhat impeded, or that the deposition or synthesis of fat was promoted; what would happen? Lack of food is the cause of hunger and, to most of the body, [fat] is the food; it is easy to imagine that a minor derangement could be responsible for a voracious appetite. It seems likely to me that hunger in the obese might be so ravaging and ravenous that skinny physicians do not understand it. . . .*

This theory would explain why dieting is so seldom effective and why most fat people are miserable when they fast. It would also take care of our friends, the psychiatrists, who find all kinds of preoccupation with food, which pervades dreams among patients who are obese. Which of us would not be preoccupied with thoughts of food if we were suffering from internal starvation? Hunger is such an awful thing that it is classically cited with pestilence and war as one of our three worst burdens. Add to the physical discomfort the emotional stresses of being fat, the taunts and

---

*In 1940, Hugo Rony described his conception of the lipophilia hypothesis in a similar manner: "Due to some anomaly of the . . . fat tissues of the obese, these tissues would remove glucose and fat from the blood faster and at lower threshold levels than normally and, when calories are needed for energy . . . would resist mobilization of fat to a greater extent than normally. In this way, increased hunger and increased caloric intake would be created, much of the consumed food being again removed by the avid fat tissues, and this process would be repeated until generalized obesity results."

teasing from the thin, the constant criticism, the accusations of gluttony and lack of "will power," and the constant guilt feelings, and we have reasons enough for the emotional disturbances which preoccupy the psychiatrists.

To understand obesity and why we get fat, we have to understand what Astwood understood and what obesity experts were beginning to accept before the Second World War put a halt to the proceedings. Both gluttony (overeating) and sloth (sedentary behavior) will be the side effects of any regulatory derangement, minor as it may be, that diverts too many calories into fat tissue for storage. Those of us so afflicted might indeed have the urge or the need to see a psychiatrist before too long. It won't be our emotional disturbances that make us fat, though, but the inexorable fattening (along with the hunger and the taunting and the accusations of gluttony and lack of "willpower") that makes us disturbed.

11

A Primer on the Regulation of Fat

It's time to roll up our sleeves and get to work. What we need to know is what biological factors regulate the amount of fat in our fat tissue. And, specifically, how this is affected by our diets, so we can know what we're doing wrong and how to change it. Another way to say this is that we need to know what determines nature—why we might be predisposed to get fat or stay lean—and what elements of nurture, of diet and lifestyle, can be altered to affect this predisposition or combat it.

I'm going to be discussing some basic biology and endocrinology, subjects you may understandably find slow going. All I can promise is that if you pay attention you'll know virtually everything you need to know about why people get fat and what has to be done to combat it.

The science I'll be talking about was worked out by researchers between the 1920s and the 1980s. At no point was it particularly controversial. Those who did the research agreed that this was how it worked, and they still agree. The problem, though, as I hope I've made clear, is that the "authorities" on obesity, even those who weren't psychologists or psychiatrists, came to believe that they knew what makes people fat—overeating and sedentary behavior. As a result, nothing else on the subject really mattered to them, including the science of how fat tissue is regulated. They either ignored it entirely or actively rejected it because they didn't like its implications (which I'll discuss later). Despite their head-in-the-sand attitude, the regulation of our fat tissue does matter. Whether we get fat or stay lean depends on it.

The Basics (Why Anyone Gets Fat)

Simple question: Why do we store fat in the first place? What's the reason? Okay, some of it provides insulation to keep us warm, and some of it provides padding to protect the more fragile structures within, but what about the rest? The fat around the waist, for instance?

The way the experts typically see it is that fat storage works as a kind of long-term savings account—like a retirement account that you can dip into only in dire need. The idea is that your body takes excess calories and stashes them away as fat, and they remain in the fat tissue until you someday find yourself sufficiently underfed (because you're now dieting or exercising or perhaps stranded on a desert island) that this fat is mobilized. You then use it for fuel.

But it has been known since the 1930s that this conception is not even remotely accurate. As it happens, fat is continuously flowing out of our fat cells and circulating around the body to be used for fuel and, if it's not used for fuel, returned to the fat cells. This goes on regardless of whether we've recently eaten or exercised. In 1948, after this science was worked out in detail, Ernst Wertheimer, a German biochemist who had emigrated to Israel and is considered the father of the field of fat metabolism, put it this way: "Mobilization and deposition of fat go on continuously, without regard to the nutritional state of the animal."*

Over the course of any twenty-four-hour period, fat from your fat cells will provide a significant portion of the fuel that your cells will burn for energy. The reason nutritionists like to think (and

---

*"Without regard to the nutritional state of the animal" is a phrase that can be found often in technical discussions of the regulation of fat tissue. It means that humans and other animals store calories as fat even when they're not eating more calories than they're expending—"even when half starved," as Jean Mayer said. As I pointed out earlier, this phrase alone makes it possible to explain the existence of obese women with starving children in impoverished societies. In

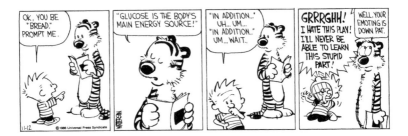

like to tell us) that carbohydrates are somehow the preferred fuel for the body, which is simply wrong, is that your cells will burn carbohydrates before they'll burn fat. They do so because that's how the body keeps blood sugar levels in check after a meal. And if you're eating a carbohydrate-rich diet, as most people do, your cells will have a lot of carbohydrates to burn before they get to the fat.

Imagine that you're eating a meal that contains both carbohydrates and fat, which most meals do. As the fat is digested, it's shipped off directly to the fat cells for storage. Think of it as being set aside temporarily while the body deals with the carbohydrates, which demand more immediate action. As these carbohydrates are digested, they appear in the bloodstream in the form of glucose, which is the "sugar" in "blood sugar." (A carbohydrate called "fructose" is a special case, and I'll discuss that later.) Cells throughout the body will burn this glucose for fuel and use it to replenish their backup fuel supplies, but they can't keep up with this rising tide of blood sugar unless they get help doing it.

This is where the hormone insulin comes in. Insulin plays many roles in the human body, but one critical role is to keep blood sugar under control. You'll start secreting insulin (from the pancreas) even before you start eating—indeed, it's stimulated

one sense, however, Wertheimer was exaggerating to make his point, because the nutritional state of the animal, as Wertheimer knew, does indeed influence the balance of mobilization and deposition—whether more fat is going in than is coming out or vice versa.

just by thinking about eating. This is a Pavlovian response. It will happen without any conscious thought. In effect, this insulin is preparing your body for the meal you're about to eat. When you take your first bites, more insulin will be secreted. And as the glucose from the meal begins flooding the circulation, still more is secreted.

The insulin then signals cells throughout the body to increase the rate at which they're pumping in glucose from the bloodstream. The cells, as I said earlier, will burn some of this glucose for immediate energy and store some for later use. Muscle cells store the glucose in the form of a molecule called "glycogen." Liver cells store some as glycogen and convert some to fat. And fat cells store it as fat.

As your blood sugar begins to decrease, and insulin levels decrease along with it, more and more of the fat stored during the meal will be released from fat tissue (or at least it should be) to take up the slack. Some of this fat began life as carbohydrates, and some began life as fat in the diet, but it's indistinguishable once it finds itself stored in the fat cells. The more time passes after a meal, the more fat you will burn and the less glucose. The reason you can sleep through the night without getting up every few hours to raid the refrigerator (or the reason you should be able to) is that fat flowing out of your fat tissue keeps your cells nicely fueled until the morning.

So the correct way to think about fat tissue is that it's more like a wallet than a savings or retirement account. You're always putting fat into it, and you're always taking fat out. You get a tiny bit fatter (more fat goes into our fat cells than comes out) during and after every meal, and then you get a tiny bit leaner again (the opposite occurs) after the meal is digested. And you get leaner still while sleeping. In an ideal world, one in which you're not getting any fatter, the calories you store as fat immediately after meals during the day are balanced out over time by the calories you burn as fat after digesting those meals and during the night.

Another way to think of this is that your fat cells work as energy buffers. They provide a place to put the calories that you consumed during a meal and don't use immediately, and then they release the calories back into the circulation as you need them — just as your wallet provides a place to put the money you withdraw from the ATM and then releases it, so to speak, as you need it throughout the day. It's only when the reserves of fat are reduced to some minimum amount that you start to get hungry again and are motivated to eat. (Just as we all have some minimum amount of cash we like to have in our wallets, and when we get down to that point, we go to the bank machine and restock.) In the early 1960s, the Swiss physiologist Albert Renold, who followed Ernst Wertheimer as the preeminent scientist in the field of fat metabolism, put it this way: our fat tissue, he wrote, is "the major site of active regulation of energy storage and mobilization, one of the primary control mechanisms responsible for the survival of any given organism."

The fact that fat is flowing into and out of our fat cells all day long, though, doesn't explain how the cells decide what fat gets to come and go, and what fat has no choice and is locked away inside. This decision is made very simply, based on the *form* of the fat. The fat in our bodies exists in two different forms that serve entirely different purposes. Fat flows in and out of cells in the form of molecules called "fatty acids"; this is also the form we *burn* for fuel. We *store* fat in the form of molecules called "triglycerides," which are composed of three fatty acids ("tri-") bound together by a molecule of glycerol ("glyceride").

The reason for this role distribution is again surprisingly simple: triglycerides are too big to flow through the membranes that surround every fat cell, whereas fatty acids are small enough to slip through cell membranes with relative ease, and so they do. Flowing back and forth, in and out of fat cells all day long, they can be burned for fuel whenever needed. Triglycerides are the form in which fat is fixed inside fat cells, stashed away for future use. For this reason, the triglycerides first have to be constructed inside a fat cell (the technical term is "esterified") from their component fatty acids, which is what happens.

When a fatty acid flows into a fat cell (or when it's created in the fat cell from scratch out of glucose), it will be bound up with a glycerol molecule and two other fatty acids, and the result is a triglyceride, a molecule now too big to get out of the fat cell. Now these three fatty acids are stuck in the fat cell until the triglyceride gets disassembled or falls apart, and they can flow out of the cell again and back into the circulation. Anyone who ever bought a piece of furniture only to realize that it's too big to fit through the door of the room for which it was intended knows the routine. You take the furniture apart (if possible), you walk the pieces through the door, and then you put the item of furniture back together on the other side. And if you move, and you want to take this particular furniture with you to your new home, you repeat the process in the other direction.

As a result, anything that works to promote the flow of fatty acids into your fat cells, where they can be bundled together into triglycerides, works to store fat, to make you fatter. Anything that

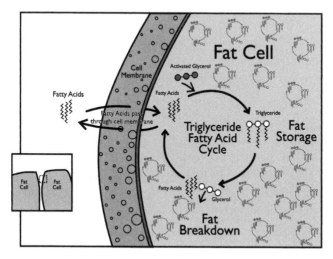

Fatty acids are small enough to flow through the membrane of the fat cell and so they do. Inside the fat cell, fatty acids are bound up as triglycerides, molecules too large to fit through the cell membrane. This is the form in which we store fat.

works to break down those triglycerides into their component fatty acids so the fatty acids can escape from the fat cells works to make you leaner. As I said, it's pretty simple. And as Edwin Astwood pointed out half a century ago, there are dozens of hormones and enzymes that play a role in these processes, and it's very easy to imagine how they can be disturbed so that too much fat gets in and not enough gets out.

One hormone dominates this action, though, and that's insulin. Astwood pointed this out almost fifty years ago, and it's never been controversial. As I said, you secrete insulin primarily in response to the carbohydrates in your diet, and you do so primarily to keep blood sugar under control.* But the insulin also works simultaneously to orchestrate the storage and use of fat and protein. It makes sure, for instance, that your muscle cells get enough protein to do whatever rebuilding and repair is necessary, and it makes sure that you store enough fuel (glycogen and fat and protein as well) to function effectively between meals. And because one place we store fuels for later use is our fat tissue, insulin is the "principal regulator of fat metabolism," which is how it was described in 1965 by Salomon Berson and Rosalyn Yalow, the two scientists who invented the technology necessary to measure hormone levels in our blood and did much of the relevant research. (Yalow later won the Nobel Prize for this work. Berson certainly would have shared it had he not died before the prize was awarded.)

Insulin accomplishes this job primarily through two enzymes. The first is LPL, lipoprotein lipase, the enzyme I discussed earlier, when we were talking about how rats get obese if their ovaries are removed. LPL is the enzyme that sticks out from the mem-

---

*Insulin is also secreted when we eat protein-rich foods, but the action is far more measured than it is for carbohydrates, and it depends in large part on the carbohydrate content of the meal. As a result, it's carbohydrates that effectively determine insulin secretion.

branes of different cells and then pulls fat out of the bloodstream and into the cells. If the LPL is on the surface of a muscle cell, then it directs the fat into the muscle to be used for fuel. If it's on a fat cell, then it makes that fat cell fatter. (The LPL breaks down triglycerides in the bloodstream into their component fatty acids, and then the fatty acids flow into the cell.) As I said previously, the female sex hormone estrogen stifles the activity of LPL on fat cells and so works to decrease fat accumulation.

LPL is the simple answer to many of the questions I raised earlier about the wheres and whens of fattening. Why do men and women fatten differently? Because the distribution of LPL is different, as is the influence of sex hormones on LPL.

In men, LPL activity is higher in the fat tissue of the gut, so this is where men tend to get fat, whereas it's low in the fat tissue below the waist. One reason men get fatter above the waist as they age is that they secrete less testosterone, a male sex hormone, and testosterone suppresses LPL activity on the abdominal fat cells. Less testosterone means more LPL activity on the fat cells of the gut, and so more fat.

In women, the activity of LPL is high on the fat cells below the waist, which is why they tend to fatten around the hips and butt, and low on the fat cells of the gut. After menopause, the LPL activity in women's abdominal fat catches up to that of men, and so they tend to put on excess fat there, too. When women get pregnant, LPL activity increases on their butts and hips; this is where they store the calories they'll need later to nurse their babies. Putting fat on below the waist and behind them also balances the weight of the child growing in their womb in front. After women give birth, the LPL activity below their waist decreases. They lose the excess fat they gained, at least most of it, but LPL activity increases in the mammary glands of their breasts, so they can use this fat to produce milk for the baby.

LPL also happens to be one very good answer to the question of why we don't lose fat when we exercise. While we're working out, LPL activity decreases on our fat cells and increases on muscle cells. This prompts the release of fat from our fat tissue, so we

can burn it in our muscle cells, which need the fuel. We get a little leaner. So far, so good. But when we're done exercising, the situation reverses. Now LPL activity on the muscle cells shuts down,
LPL activity on the fat cells shoots up, and the fat cells restock
whatever fat they lost during the workout. We get fatter again.
(This also explains why exercise makes us hungry. Not only do
our muscles crave protein after a workout to restock and rebuild,
but our fat is actively restocking, too. The rest of the body tries to
compensate for this energy drain, and our appetite increases.)

Since insulin is the primary regulator of fat metabolism, it's
not surprising that it's the primary regulator of LPL activity.
Insulin activates LPL on fat cells, particularly the fat cells of the
abdomen; it "upregulates" LPL, as researchers say. The more
insulin we secrete, the more active the LPL on the fat cells, and
the more fat is diverted from the bloodstream into the fat cells to
be stored. Insulin also happens to suppress LPL activity on the
muscle cells, assuring that they won't have many fatty acids to
burn. (Insulin also tells muscle cells and others in the body *not* to
burn fatty acids but to continue burning up blood sugar instead.)
This means that when fatty acids do escape from a fat cell, if
insulin levels happen to be high, these fatty acids won't be taken
up by the muscle cells and used for fuel. They'll end up back in
the fat tissue.*

Insulin also influences an enzyme that we haven't discussed,
hormone-sensitive lipase, or HSL for short. And this may be even
more critical to how insulin regulates the amount of fat we store.
Just as LPL works to make fat cells (and us) fatter, HSL works to
make fat cells (and us) leaner. It does so by working inside the fat
cells to break down triglycerides into their component fatty acids,
so that those fatty acids can then escape into the circulation. The
more active this HSL, the more fat we liberate and can burn for
fuel and the less, obviously, we store. Insulin also suppresses this

---

*Here is a technical description from the 2008 edition of *Williams Textbook
of Endocrinology*: "Insulin influences [the partitioning of triglycerides among
different body tissues] through its stimulation of LPL activity in adipose tissue."

enzyme HSL, and so it prevents triglycerides from being broken down inside the fat cells and keeps the outward flow of fatty acids from the fat cells to a minimum. And it takes just a little bit of insulin to accomplish this feat of shutting down HSL and trapping fat in our fat cells. When insulin levels are elevated, even a little, fat accumulates in the fat cells.

Insulin also turns on a mechanism in the fat cells to pump in glucose—just as it does in muscle cells—and this increases the amount of glucose the fat cells metabolize. This in turn increases the amount of glycerol molecules (a by-product of glucose metabolism) floating around in the fat cells, and these glycerol molecules can now be bundled together with fatty acids into triglycerides, and so more fat can be stored. To assure we have room to store all that fat, insulin also works to create new fat cells in case the ones we already have are getting full. And insulin signals liver cells not to burn fatty acids but to repackage them into triglycerides and ship them back to the fat tissue. It even triggers the conversion of carbohydrates directly into fatty acids in the liver and in the fat tissue, although how much this actually goes on in humans (as opposed to lab rats) is still a subject of debate.

In short, everything insulin does in this context works to increase the fat we store and decrease the fat we burn. Insulin works to make us fatter.

The photo on page 122 shows a particularly graphic example of this fattening effect of insulin, courtesy of the textbook *Endocrinology: An Integrated Approach* by Stephen Nussly and Saffron Whitehead, which the National Library of Medicine makes available online (http://www.ncbi.nlm.nih.gov/bookshelf/br.fcgi?book=endocrin). The caption of this photo is "The effects of insulin on adipose tissue."

The woman pictured developed type 1 diabetes when she was seventeen. The photo was taken forty-seven years later. In the intervening years, she faithfully injected herself with her daily insulin in the same two sites on her thighs. The result:

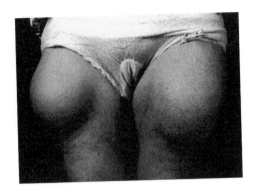

cantaloupe-sized masses of fat on each thigh. And these obviously have nothing to do with how much she ate, only the fattening or "lipogenic" effect of the insulin. Keep in mind that it took this woman decades to amass these unsightly fat deposits. For her, it would have seemed barely noticeable year to year, just as it does for many of us when we get fat.

When we raise insulin levels throughout our body, this is what happens. This is why diabetics often get fatter when they take insulin therapy. (It results from "the direct lipogenic effect of insulin on adipose tissue, independent of food intake," as explained by the seminal textbook in the field, *Joslin's Diabetes Mellitus*.) In one study published in *The New England Journal of Medicine* in 2008, type 2 diabetics on intensive insulin therapy gained an average of eight pounds, and almost one in every three of these diabetics gained more than twenty pounds in three and a half years.

Because the insulin level in the bloodstream is determined primarily by the carbohydrates that are consumed—their quantity and quality, as I'll discuss—*it's those carbohydrates that ultimately determine how much fat we accumulate.* Here's the chain of events:

1. You think about eating a meal containing carbohydrates.
2. You begin secreting insulin.

3. The insulin signals the fat cells to shut down the release of fatty acids (by inhibiting HSL) and take up more fatty acids (via LPL) from the circulation.
4. You start to get hungry, or hungrier.
5. You begin eating.
6. You secrete more insulin.
7. The carbohydrates are digested and enter the circulation as glucose, causing blood sugar levels to rise.*
8. You secrete still more insulin.
9. Fat from the diet is stored as triglycerides in the fat cells, as are some of the carbohydrates that are converted into fat in the liver.
10. The fat cells get fatter, and so do you.
11. The fat stays in the fat cells until the insulin level drops.

If you're wondering whether any other hormones make us fat, the answer is effectively no, with one significant exception.†

One way to think about what hormones do is that they instruct the body to do something—grow and develop (growth hormones), reproduce (sex hormones), flee or fight (adrenaline). They also make the fuel available for those various actions. Among other things, they signal our fat tissue to mobilize fatty acids and make them available for fuel.

For example, we secrete adrenaline in response to perceived threats. It readies us to flee or fight should the need arise. But if you had to flee a charging lion, say, and you didn't have the fuel immediately available to run either faster or farther (and maybe both) than the lion, the lion would catch you. So, on seeing the

---

*Once again, this doesn't include fructose, a special case, as I will soon discuss.

†A hormone discovered in the late 1980s known as acylation stimulating protein is almost assuredly an insignificant exception. It is secreted by the fat tissue itself, a process that is regulated at least in part by insulin.

lion, you secrete adrenaline, and the adrenaline, among other things, signals your fat tissue to dump fatty acids into the circulation. These fatty acids, ideally, will then provide all the fuel you need to make your escape. In this sense, every hormone but insulin works to release fat from our fat tissue. They make us leaner, at least temporarily.

These other hormones, though, have a far more difficult time getting fat out of fat tissue if the insulin level in the circulation is elevated. Insulin trumps the effect of other hormones. It's all very rational. If there's a lot of insulin around, it *should* mean there are also a lot of carbohydrates around to burn—that the blood sugar level is high—and so we don't need or want fatty acids getting in the way. As a result, these other hormones will liberate fat from the fat tissue only when insulin levels are low. (The other hormones work by stimulating HSL to break down triglycerides, but the HSL is so sensitive to insulin that the other hormones can't overcome its action.)

The one meaningful exception is cortisol. This is the hormone we secrete in response to stress or anxiety. Cortisol actually works to put fat into our fat tissue *and* to get it out. It puts fat in by stimulating the enzyme LPL, just as insulin does, and by causing or exacerbating a condition known as "insulin resistance," which I'll discuss in the next chapter. When you're insulin-resistant, you secrete more insulin and you store more fat.

So cortisol makes us store fat both directly (through LPL) and indirectly (through insulin). But then it works to release fat from our fat cells, primarily by stimulating HSL, just like other hormones. So cortisol can make us fatter still when insulin is elevated, but it can also make us leaner, just like every other hormone, when insulin levels are low. And this may explain why some people get fatter when they get stressed, anxious, or depressed and eat more, and some people do the opposite.

The bottom line is something that's been known (and mostly ignored) for over forty years. The one thing we absolutely have to do if we want to get leaner—if we want to get fat out of our fat tissue and burn it—is to lower our insulin levels and to secrete less insulin to begin with. Here's how Yalow and Berson phrased it back in 1965: releasing fat from our fat tissue and then burning it for energy, they wrote, "requires only the negative stimulus of insulin deficiency." If we can get our insulin levels to drop sufficiently low (the negative stimulus of insulin deficiency), we can burn our fat. If we can't, we won't. When we secrete insulin, or if the level of insulin in our blood is abnormally elevated, we'll accumulate fat in the fat tissue. That's what the science tells us.

The Implications

Earlier I talked about the twenty-four-hour cycle of storing and burning fat. We gain it during the day, when we're digesting meals (because of the effects of carbohydrates on insulin); we lose it in the hours until our next meal, and at night, while we're sleeping. Ideally, the fat we gain during the fat-storage phases is balanced by the fat we lose during the fat-burning phases. What we gain during the day is burned during the night, and it's insulin that ultimately controls this cycle. As I've said, when insulin levels go up, we store fat. When they come down, we mobilize the fat and use it for fuel.

This suggests that anything that makes us secrete more insulin than nature intended, or keeps insulin levels elevated for longer than nature intended, will extend the periods during which we store fat and shorten the periods when we burn it. As we know, the imbalance that results—more fat stored, less burned—can border on infinitesimal, twenty calories a day, and it can lead us to obesity within a couple of decades.*

By extending the periods when we're storing fat rather than

---

*In 1984, a brilliant French physiologist named Jacques Le Magnen described the situation this way: "It is not a paradox," he wrote, "to say that animals and humans that become obese gain weight because they are no longer able to lose weight."

burning it, insulin indirectly has another effect. Remember, we depend on fatty acids for fuel in the hours after a meal, as blood sugar levels are dropping to their pre-meal level. But the insulin suppresses the flow of fatty acid from the fat cells; it tells the other cells in the body to burn carbohydrates. So, as blood sugar returns to a healthy level, we need a replacement fuel supply.

If insulin remains elevated, the fat isn't available. Nor is protein, which our cells can also use for fuel if necessary: insulin also works to keep the protein stored away in the muscles. We can't use the carbohydrates we've stored in the liver and muscle tissue, either, because the insulin keeps that supply locked up as well.

As a result, the cells find themselves starved for fuel, and we quite literally feel *their* hunger. Either we eat sooner than we otherwise would have or we eat more when we do eat, or both. As I said earlier, anything that makes us fatter will make us overeat in the process. That's what insulin does.

Meanwhile, our bodies are getting bigger because we're putting on fat, and so our fuel requirements are increasing. When we get fatter, we also add muscle to support that fat. (Thanks again in part to insulin, which assures that whatever protein we consume is used for repairing muscle cells and organs and for adding muscle, if necessary.) So, as we fatten, our energy demand increases, and our appetite will increase for this reason as well— particularly our appetite for carbohydrates, because this is the only nutrient our cells will burn for fuel when insulin is elevated. This is a vicious cycle, and it's precisely what we'd like to avoid. If we're predisposed to get fat, we'll be driven to crave precisely those carbohydrate-rich foods that make us fat.

12

Why I Get Fat and You Don't (or Vice Versa)

If insulin makes people fat, why does it make only some of us fat? We all secrete insulin, after all, and yet plenty of us are lean and will stay lean for life. This is a question of nature—our genetic predisposition—not nurture or the aspects of diet and/or lifestyle that trigger this nature.

The answer lies in the fact that hormones don't work in a vacuum, and insulin is no exception. The effect of a hormone on any particular tissue or cell depends on a host of factors, both inside and outside cells—on enzymes, for instance, such as LPL and HSL. This allows hormones to differ in their effect from cell to cell, tissue to tissue, and even at different stages of our development and our lives.

One way to think about insulin in this context is as a hormone that determines how fuels are "partitioned" around the body. After a meal, insulin and the various enzymes it influences, such as LPL, determine what proportion of the different nutrients will be sent to which tissues, how much will be burned, how much will be stored, and how this will change with need and with time. Since I'm concerned here with whether fuels will be used for energy or stored, imagine insulin and these enzymes as determining which way the needle points on what I'm going to call a fuel-partitioning gauge. Imagine it looking like the fuel gauge in your car, but instead of the "F" standing for "full" on the right, it stands for "fat," and the "E" on the left doesn't stand for "empty," but for "energy."

If the needle points to the right—toward the "F"—it means that insulin partitions a disproportionate amount of the calories you consume into storage as fat, rather than use for energy by the muscles. In this case, you'll have a tendency to fatten, and you'll have less energy available for physical activity, so you'll also tend to be sedentary. The farther the needle points toward fat storage, the more calories will be stored, the fatter you'll be. If you don't want to be sedentary, of course, then you have to eat more to compensate for this loss of calories into fat.* It's the morbidly obese people of the world who live on the far end of this side of the gauge.

When the needle points in the other direction—toward the "E"—you'll be burning as fuel a disproportionate share of the calories you consume. You'll have plenty of energy for physical activity, but little will be stored as fat. You'll be lean and active (just as you're supposed to be), and you'll eat in moderation. The farther out you go in this direction, the more energy you'll have for physical activity and the less will be stored—the leaner you'll be. Emaciated-looking marathoners can be found down here. Their bodies burn calories—they don't store them—and so these people literally have energy to burn. They have what pre–World War II metabolism researchers would have called a very powerful impulse to be physically active.

What determines the direction in which the needle points? The answer is not quite as simple as how much insulin you secrete, although that's probably part of it. Given the same food containing the same amount of carbohydrates, some people will

---

*To be precise, the insulin stashes fat in the fat tissue and assures that it stays there. Our muscles are forced to burn more carbohydrates to compensate, and we deplete our reserves of glycogen, which alone might make us hungrier. The result is that we want to eat more and expend less, while our fat tissue just keeps filling up with fat.

secrete more insulin than others, and those who do are likely to put on more fat and have less energy. Their bodies work to keep blood sugar levels under control, because high blood sugar is toxic, and they're willing to overstuff their fat cells, if necessary, to do it.

But another important factor is just how sensitive to insulin your cells happen to be and how quickly they become insensitive—the property called "insulin resistance"—in response to the insulin you secrete. This idea of being resistant to insulin is absolutely critical to understanding the reasons we get fat and also many of the diseases associated with it. I'll return to it frequently.

The more insulin you secrete, the more likely it is that your cells and tissues will become resistant to that insulin. That means it will take more insulin to do the same glucose-disposal job, keeping blood sugar under control. One way to think about it is that your cells make the decision that they don't want any more glucose than they're already getting—too much glucose is toxic for cells, too—so they make it harder for insulin to do its job and get the glucose out of the bloodstream.

The problem (or the solution, depending on point of view) is that the pancreas responds by pumping out still more insulin. And the result is a vicious cycle. When a lot of insulin is secreted—in response to easily digestible carbohydrates, say—your cells are likely to resist the effects of that insulin, at least in the short term, particularly your muscle cells, because they're getting enough glucose already. If these cells become resistant to insulin, more insulin is required to keep blood sugar levels in check, so now you secrete more insulin, which prompts more insulin resistance. And all the while, that insulin is working to make you fatter (to store calories as fat), unless your fat cells are also resistant to it.

So secreting more insulin will move the needle on the fuel-partitioning gauge toward storage. But if you secrete a healthy amount of insulin, and yet your muscle tissue is relatively quick to become resistant to that insulin, you'll achieve the same thing.

You'll secrete more insulin in response to the insulin resistance, and you'll grow fatter.

A third factor is that your cells will respond differently to insulin. Fat cells, muscle cells, liver cells don't all become resistant to insulin at the same time, to the same extent, or in the same way. Some of these cells will become more or less sensitive to insulin than others, which means the same amount of insulin will have a greater or lesser effect on different tissues. And how these tissues respond will differ as well—from person to person and, as I'll discuss, over time in the same individual.

The more sensitive a particular tissue is to insulin, the more glucose it will take up when insulin is secreted. If it's muscle, it will store more glucose as glycogen and burn more for fuel. If it's fat, it will store more fat and release less. So, if your muscle cells are very sensitive to insulin and your fat cells less so, then the needle of the fuel-partitioning gauge points toward fuel burning. Your muscles will take up a disproportionate share of the glucose from the carbohydrates you consume, and they'll use it for energy. The result: you'll be lean and physically active. If your muscles are relatively insensitive to insulin compared with your fat cells, then your fat tissue will be the repository of a disproportionate share of the calories you consume. As a result, you'll be fat and sedentary.*

Here's another complication: how your tissues respond to insulin changes will change with time (and in response to your diet, as I'll discuss shortly). As you get older, you get more insulin-resistant,

---

* The effect of making particular tissues insulin-resistant can be mimicked in laboratory mice and has been by researchers at the Joslin Diabetes Center in Boston. They created mice that lack what are called insulin "receptors" on different tissues, which means those tissues are completely resistant to insulin. As we'd expect, mice that lack insulin receptors on their muscle cells but not on their fat cells get obese. The animals partition glucose into the fat for storage, not the muscles for energy. Mice that lack insulin receptors on their fat cells are lean, and they stay lean, even when they're force-fed more food than they'd otherwise prefer to eat.

but this almost invariably happens to your muscle tissue first and only later, if at all, to your fat tissue. As a general rule, fat cells always stay more sensitive to insulin than muscle cells do. So, even if you're lean and active when you're young, with your fuel-partitioning needle pointing toward fuel burning, your muscle cells are likely to become resistant to insulin as you get older. As they do, you'll respond by secreting more insulin.

This means the needle on the fuel-partitioning gauge will move to the right as you age—more and more calories will be diverted into fat, leaving fewer and fewer available to fuel the rest of the body. As you enter middle age, you'll find it increasingly difficult to remain lean. You'll also begin to manifest a multitude of other metabolic disturbances that accompany this insulin resistance and the elevated insulin levels that go hand in hand: your blood pressure goes up, as does your triglyceride level; your HDL cholesterol (aka, the "good cholesterol") goes down; you become glucose intolerant, which means you have trouble controlling your blood sugar, and so on. And you'll become increasingly sedentary, a side effect of the energy drain into the fat tissue.

In fact, the conventional wisdom that those of us who fatten as we move into middle age do so because our metabolism slows down, probably has this cause and effect backward. More likely is that our muscles become increasingly resistant to insulin, and this partitions more of the energy we consume into fat, leaving less available for the cells of muscles and organs to use for fuel. These cells now generate less energy, and this is what we mean when we say that our metabolism slows down. Our "metabolic rate" decreases. Once again, what appears to be a cause of fattening—the slowing of our metabolism—is really an effect. You don't get fat because your metabolism slows; your metabolism slows because you're getting fat.

Before I discuss the nurture side of this issue, the foods we eat that make things worse and that we can live without, there is one more issue of nature to discuss: why our children are today getting fatter, and maybe even coming out of the womb fatter, than just twenty or thirty years ago. This is one aspect of the obesity epidemic that's emerged recently in studies worldwide. Not only are more children obese now than ever before, but most studies report that they're noticeably fatter at six months, a phenomenon that obviously has nothing to do with their behavior.

Fat children tend to be born of fat parents, in part because of all the ways that our genes control our insulin secretion, the enzymes that respond to insulin, and how and when we become resistant to insulin. But there's also another factor that represents cause for concern. Children in the womb are supplied with nutrients from the mother (through the placenta and umbilical cord) in proportion to the level of those nutrients in the mother's blood. This means that the higher the level of the mother's blood sugar, the more glucose her child gets in her womb.

As the pancreas in that child develops, it apparently responds to this higher dose of glucose by developing more insulin-secreting cells. So, the higher the blood sugar in the pregnant mother, the more insulin-secreting cells her child will develop, and the more insulin the child will secrete as it gets close to birth. The baby will now be born with more fat, and it will have a tendency to oversecrete insulin and become insulin-resistant itself as it gets older. It will be predisposed to get fat as it ages. In animal studies, this predisposition often manifests itself only when the animal reaches its version of middle age. If this observation translates to humans, then some of us are programmed in the womb to get fat in middle age, even if we show little or no sign of this predisposition when we're young.

This is almost assuredly the reason why obese mothers, diabetic mothers, mothers who gain excessive weight during pregnancy, and mothers who become diabetic in pregnancy (a condition known as "gestational diabetes") all tend to have larger and fatter babies. These women tend to be insulin-resistant and have high levels of blood sugar.

But if fatter mothers have fatter babies, and fatter babies

become fatter mothers, where does it stop? This suggests that, as the obesity epidemic took off, and we all began getting fatter, we began to program more and more of our children from the first few months of their existence to get fatter still. In fact, it wouldn't be surprising if this particular vicious cycle is one cause of the obesity epidemic. Thus we have more than our own health to consider when we get fat. Our children, too, may pay a price, and their children. And each successive generation may find it that much harder to undo the problem.

13

What We Can Do

Whether you're born predisposed to get fat is beyond your control. What Adiposity 101 teaches us, though, is that this predisposition is set off by the carbohydrates we eat—by their quantity and their quality. As I said, it's carbohydrates that ultimately determines insulin secretion and insulin that drives the accumulation of body fat. Not all of us get fat when we eat carbohydrates, but for those of us who do get fat, the carbohydrates are to blame; the fewer carbohydrates we eat, the leaner we will be.

A comparison with cigarettes is apt. Not every longtime smoker gets lung cancer. Only one in six men will, and one in nine women. But for those who do get lung cancer, cigarette smoke is far and away the most common cause. In a world without cigarettes, lung cancer would be a rare disease, as it once was. In a world without carbohydrate-rich diets, obesity would be a rare condition as well.

Not that all foods that contain carbohydrates are equally fattening. This is a crucial point. The most fattening foods are the ones that have the greatest effect on our blood sugar and insulin levels. These are the concentrated sources of carbohydrates, and particularly those that we can digest quickly: anything made of refined flour (bread, cereals, and pasta), liquid carbohydrates (beers, fruit juices, and sodas), and starches (potatoes, rice, and corn). These foods flood the bloodstream quickly with glucose. Blood sugar shoots up; insulin shoots up. We get fatter. Not surprisingly, these foods have been considered uniquely fattening for nearly two hundred years (as I'll discuss later).*

These foods are also, almost invariably, the cheapest calories available. This is the conspicuous explanation for why the poorer we are, the fatter we're likely to be; why, as I discussed at the outset, it's all too easy to find extremely poor populations, past and present, with obesity and diabetes rates that rival those in the United States and Europe today. This was the explanation suggested by physicians who worked with these populations in the 1960s and 1970s, and now we know it's supported by the science.

"Most third world countries have a high carbohydrate intake," wrote Rolf Richards, the British-turned-Jamaican diabetes specialist in 1974. "It is conceivable that the ready availability of starch in preference to animal protein, contributing as it must the main caloric requirements of these populations, leads to increased lipogenesis [fat formation] and the development of obesity." People in these populations get fat not because they eat too much or are too sedentary but because the foods they live on—the starches and refined grains that make up the great majority of their diet, and the sugar—are literally fattening.

The carbohydrates in leafy green vegetables like spinach and kale, on the other hand, are bound up with indigestible fiber and take much longer to be digested and enter our bloodstream. These vegetables contain more water and fewer digestible carbohydrates for their weight than starches like potatoes. We have to eat far more to get the same load of carbohydrates, and those carbohydrates take longer to digest. As a result, blood sugar levels remain relatively low when we eat these vegetables; they initiate a

---

*How our blood sugar responds to different foods is known technically as the "glycemic index," a reasonably good measure of how our insulin will respond. The higher the glycemic index of a particular food, the greater the blood sugar response. Entire books have been published on the idea of minimizing the glycemic index of our diets and, by doing so, minimizing the insulin we secrete and the fat we accumulate.

far more modest insulin response and are therefore less fattening. It is possible, though, that some people may be so sensitive to the carbohydrates in their diet that even these green vegetables may be a problem.

The carbohydrates in fruits, though relatively easy to digest, are also diluted more by water and so are less concentrated than the carbohydrates in starches. Given an apple and a potato of the same weight, the potato will have a significantly greater effect on blood sugar, which suggests that it *should* be more fattening. But that doesn't mean fruit won't fatten some people.

What makes fruit worrisome from the perspective of Adiposity 101 is that it is sweet to the taste precisely because it contains a type of sugar known as fructose, and fructose is uniquely fattening as carbohydrates go. As nutritionists and public-health authorities have become increasingly desperate in their attempts to rein in the obesity epidemic, they've also become increasingly strident in their suggestions that we eat copious fruit along with green vegetables. Fruit doesn't have to be processed before we eat it: it's fat- and cholesterol-free; it has vitamins (vitamin C in particular) and antioxidants; and so, by this logic, it must be good for us. Maybe so. But if we're predisposed to put on fat, it's a good bet that most fruit will make the problem worse, not better.

The very worst foods for us, almost assuredly, are indeed sugars—sucrose (table sugar) and high-fructose corn syrup in particular. Public-health authorities and journalists have recently taken to attacking high-fructose corn syrup as a cause of the obesity epidemic. It was introduced in 1978 and replaced the sugar in most soft drinks in the United States by the mid-1980s. Total sugar consumption ("caloric sweeteners," as the Department of Agriculture calls them, to distinguish them from "non-caloric" artificial sweeteners) promptly increased from roughly 120 pounds per capita yearly to 150, since Americans didn't realize that high-fructose corn syrup was just another form of sugar. It is, though. I'm going to refer to both of them as sugars, because they are effectively identical. Sucrose, the white granulated stuff we put in our coffee and sprinkle on our cereal, is half fructose and half glucose. High-fructose corn syrup, in the form we typically get it in juices, sodas, and fruity yogurts, is 55 percent fructose (which is why it's known in the food industry as HFCS-55) 42 percent glucose, and 3 percent other carbohydrates.

It's the fructose in these sweeteners that makes them sweet, just as it makes fruit sweet, and it appears to be the fructose that makes them so fattening and, in turn, so bad for our health. The American Heart Association and other authorities have lately—better late than never—taken to targeting fructose, and thus sugar and high-fructose corn syrup, as a cause of obesity and maybe even heart disease, but they do so primarily on the basis that these sweeteners are "empty calories," which means they don't come with any vitamins, minerals, or antioxidants attached. This misses the point, however. Fructose actually has unhealthy effects—including making us fat—that have little to do with its lack of vitamins or antioxidants and far more to do with how our bodies process it. The sugary combination of roughly half fructose and half glucose might be particularly effective in making us fat.

When we digest the carbohydrates in starches, they eventually enter our bloodstream as glucose. Blood sugar increases, insulin is secreted, and calories are stored as fat. When we digest sugar or high-fructose corn syrup, much of the glucose ends up in the general circulation, raising our blood sugar levels. The fructose, however, is metabolized almost exclusively in the liver, which has the necessary enzymes to do it. So fructose has no immediate effect on our blood sugar and insulin levels, but the key word is "immediate"—it has plenty of long-term effects.

The human body, and particularly the liver, never evolved to handle the kind of fructose load we get in modern diets. Fructose exists in fruits in relatively small quantities—thirty calories in a cup of blueberries, for instance. (Some fruit, though, as I'll discuss later, has been bred for generations to increase its fructose content.) There are eighty calories' worth in a twelve-ounce can of Pepsi or Coke. Twelve ounces of apple juice has eighty-five calories of fructose. Our livers respond to this flood of fructose by turning much of it into fat and shipping it to our fat tissue. This is why even forty years ago biochemists referred to fructose as the most "lipogenic" carbohydrate—it's the one we convert to fat most readily. Meanwhile, the glucose that comes with the fructose raises blood sugar levels and stimulates insulin secretion and puts the fat cells in the mode to store whatever calories come their way—including the fat generated in the liver from the fructose.

The more of these sugars we consume, and the longer we have them in our diet, the more our bodies apparently adapt by converting them to fat. Our "pattern of fructose metabolism" changes with time, as the British biochemist and fructose expert Peter Mayes says. Not only will this cause us to accumulate fat directly in the liver—a condition known as "fatty liver disease"—but it apparently causes our muscle tissue to become resistant to insulin through a kind of domino effect that is triggered by the liver cells' resistance.

So, even though fructose has no immediate effect on blood sugar and insulin, over time—maybe a few years—it is a likely cause of insulin resistance and thus the increased storage of calories as fat. The needle on our fuel-partitioning gauge will point toward fat storage, even if it didn't start out that way.

It's quite possible that if we never ate these sugars we might never become fat or diabetic, even if the bulk of our diet were still starchy carbohydrates and flour. This would explain why some of the world's poorest populations live on carbohydrate-rich diets and don't get fat or diabetic, while others aren't so lucky. The ones that don't (or at least didn't), like the Japanese and Chinese, were the ones that traditionally ate very little sugar. Once you do start to fatten, if you want to stop the process and reverse it, these sugars have to be the first to go.

Alcohol is a special case. Alcohol is metabolized mostly in the liver. Some 80 percent of the calories from a shot of vodka, for instance, will go straight to the liver to be converted into a small amount of energy and a large amount of a molecule called "citrate." The citrate then fuels the process that makes fatty acids out of glucose. So alcohol will increase the production of fat in the liver, which probably explains alcoholic fatty liver syndrome. It might also make us fatter elsewhere, although whether we store these fats as fat or burn them might depend on whether we eat or drink carbohydrates with the alcohol, which we usually do. Roughly a third of the calories in a typical beer, for instance, come originally from maltose—a refined carbohydrate—compared with the two-thirds from the alcohol itself. A beer belly is the conspicuous result.

14

Injustice Collecting

The message of Adiposity 101 is simple enough: if you're predisposed to get fat and want to be as lean as you can be without compromising your health, you have to restrict carbohydrates and so keep your blood sugar and insulin levels low. The point to keep in mind is that you don't lose fat because you cut calories; you lose fat because you cut out the foods that make you fat—the carbohydrates. If you get down to a weight you like and then add these foods back to the diet, you'll get fat again. That only some people get fat from eating carbohydrates (just as only some get lung cancer from smoking cigarettes) doesn't change the fact that if you're one of those who do, you'll only lose fat and keep it off if you avoid these foods.

This isn't the only injustice involved here. It's not even the worst of them. As I said in the introduction, the implications of Adiposity 101 do not include the ability to lose weight or maintain it without sacrifice. So far, the message is that carbohydrates make us fat and keep us fat. But the precise foods responsible for making us fat are also the ones we're likely to rank highest on a list of foods we crave and would never want to live without—pasta, bagels, bread, French fries, sweets, and beer among them.

This is not a coincidence. It's clear from animal research that the foods animals will preferentially eat perhaps to excess are those that most quickly supply energy to the cells—easily digestible carbohydrates.

But another factor is how hungry we are, which is another way of saying how long it's been since our last meal and how much energy we've expended in the interim. The longer we go between meals and the more energy we've expended, the hungrier we'll be. And the hungrier we are, the better foods will taste: *Wow! That was great. I was starving.* "It is often said and not without reason," as Pavlov wrote more than a century ago, "that 'hunger is the best sauce.'"

Even before we begin eating, insulin works to increase our feeling of hunger. Remember, we begin secreting insulin just by thinking about eating (and particularly eating carbohydrate-rich foods and sweets), and this insulin secretion then increases within seconds of taking our first bite. It happens even before we begin to digest the meal, and before any glucose appears in the bloodstream. This insulin serves to prepare our bodies for the upcoming flood of glucose by storing away other nutrients in the circulation — particularly fatty acids. So our experience of hunger actually increases just by thinking about eating, and then it increases further with the first few bites we take. (The French have a saying for this: *"L'appétit vient en mangeant,"* the appetite comes while eating.)

As the meal continues, this "metabolic background of hunger," as the French scientist Jacques Le Magnen called it, begins to ebb, our appetite is satisfied, and our perception of the palatability of the meal, how good it tastes, diminishes as well. The insulin is now working in the brain to suppress appetite and eating behavior. As a result, our first bites of a meal will invariably taste better to us than our last bites. (This is why the phrase "good to the last bite" is used to describe a product or experience that is particularly tasty or enjoyable.) This is the likely physiological explanation for why so many of us — fat or lean — become so fond of pasta and bagels and other carbohydrate-rich foods. Just by thinking about eating them, we secrete insulin. The insulin makes us hungry by temporarily diverting nutrients out of the circulation and into storage, and this, in turn, makes us savor our first bites even more than we otherwise would. The greater the blood sugar and insulin response to a particular food, the more we like it—the better we think it tastes.

This palatability-by-blood-sugar-and-insulin response is almost assuredly exaggerated in people who are fat or predisposed to get that way. And the fatter they get, the more they'll crave carbohydrate-rich foods, because their insulin will be more effective at stashing fat and protein in their muscle and fat tissue, where they can't be used for fuel.

Once we get resistant to insulin, which will happen eventually, we'll have more insulin coursing through our veins during much, if not all, of the day. Hence, we'll also have longer periods during every twenty-four hours when the only fuel we can burn is the glucose from carbohydrates. The insulin, remember, is working to keep protein and fat and even glycogen (the storage form of carbohydrates) safely stashed away for later. It's telling our cells that there is blood sugar in excess to be burned, but there's *not*. So it's glucose we crave. Even if you eat fat and protein—a hamburger without the bun, say, or a hunk of cheese—the insulin will work to store these nutrients rather than allow your body to burn them for fuel. You will have little desire to eat it, at least not without some carbohydrate-rich bread as well, because your body, at the moment, has little interest in burning it for fuel.

Sweets, again, are a special case, which probably won't be a surprise to anyone with a sweet tooth (or anyone who's ever raised a child). First, the unique metabolic effects of fructose in the liver, combined with the insulin-stimulating effect of glucose, might be enough to induce cravings in those predisposed to fatten. But then there's the effect in the brain: when you eat sugar, according to research by Bartley Hoebel of Princeton University, it triggers a response in the same part of the brain—known as the "reward center"—that is targeted by cocaine, alcohol, nicotine, and other addictive substances. All food does this to some extent, because that's what the reward system apparently evolved to do: reinforce behaviors (eating and sex) that benefit the species. But sugar seems to hijack the signal to an unnatural degree, just as cocaine and nicotine do. If we believe the animal research, then sugar and high-fructose corn syrup are addictive in the same way that drugs are and for much the same biochemical reasons.*

Now, how's that for a vicious cycle? The foods that make us fat also make us crave precisely the foods that make us fat. (This, again, is little different from smoking: the cigarettes that give us lung cancer also make us crave the cigarettes that give us lung cancer.) The more fattening they are, and the more predisposed you are to get fat when you eat them, the greater the cravings. The cycle can be broken, although it requires fighting these cravings—just as alcoholics can quit drinking and smokers can quit smoking, but not without constant effort and vigilance.

*Even cattle can be induced to eat foods they otherwise disdain by "sugar-coating" them, as researchers reported in the *Journal of Range Management* back in 1952.

15

Why Diets Succeed and Fail

The simple answer to the question of why we get fat is that carbohydrates make us so; protein and fat do not. But if this is the case, why do we all know people who have gone on low-fat diets and lost weight? Low-fat diets, after all, are relatively high in carbohydrates, so shouldn't these fail for all the people who try them?

Most of us know people who say they lost significant weight after joining Weight Watchers or Jenny Craig, after reading *Skinny Bitch* or *French Women Don't Get Fat,* or following the very low-fat diet prescribed by Dean Ornish in *Eat More, Weigh Less.* When researchers test the effectiveness of diets in clinical trials, like the Stanford University A TO Z Trial that I'll discuss shortly, they'll invariably find that a few subjects do indeed lose considerable weight following low-fat diets. Doesn't this mean that some of us get fat because we eat carbohydrates and get lean again when we don't, but for others, avoiding fat is the answer?

The simple answer is probably not. The more likely explanation is that any diet that succeeds does so because the dieter restricts fattening carbohydrates, whether by explicit instruction or not. To put it simply, those who lose fat on a diet do so because of what they are not eating—the fattening carbohydrates—not because of what they are eating.

Whenever we go on any serious weight-loss regimen, whether a diet or an exercise program, we invariably make a few consistent changes to what we eat, regardless of the instructions we're given. Specifically, we rid the diet of the most fattening of the carbohydrates, because these are the easiest to eliminate and the most obviously inappropriate if we're trying to get in shape. We stop drinking beer, for instance, or at least we drink less, or drink light beer instead. We might think of this as cutting calories, but the calories we're cutting are carbohydrates, and, more important, they're liquid, refined carbohydrates, which are exceedingly fattening.

We'll stop drinking caloric sodas—Coca-Cola, Pepsi, Dr Pepper—and replace them with either water or diet sodas. In doing so, we're not just removing the liquid carbohydrates that constitute the calories but the fructose, which is specifically responsible for making the sodas sweet. The same is true of fruit juices. An easy change in any diet is to replace fruit juices with water. We'll get rid of candy bars, desserts, donuts, and cinnamon buns. Again, we'll perceive this as calorie cutting—and maybe even a way to cut fat, which it can be—but we're also cutting carbohydrates, specifically fructose. (Even the very low-fat diet made famous by Dean Ornish restricts all refined carbohydrates, including sugar, white rice, and white flour.* This alone could explain any benefits that result.) Starches like potatoes and rice, refined carbohydrates like bread and pasta, will often be replaced by green vegetables, salads, or at least whole grains, because we've been told for the past few decades to eat more fiber and to eat foods that are less energy-dense.

If we try to cut any significant number of calories from our diet, we'll be cutting the total amount of carbohydrates we consume as well. This is just arithmetic. If we cut all the calories we consume by half, for instance, then we're cutting the carbohydrates by half, too. And because carbohydrates constitute the largest proportion of calories in our diet, these will see the greatest

---

*Ornish's rationale, as he described it in 1996: "Simple carbohydrates are absorbed quickly and cause a rapid rise in serum glucose, thereby provoking an insulin response. Insulin also accelerates conversion of calories into triglycerides, [and] stimulates . . . cholesterol synthesis."

absolute reduction. Even if our goal is to cut fat calories, we'll find it exceedingly difficult to cut more than a few hundred calories a day by reducing fat, and so we'll have to eat fewer carbohydrates as well. Low-fat diets that also cut calories will cut carbohydrates by as much or more.*

Simply put, any time we try to diet by any of the conventional methods, and any time we decide to "eat healthy" as it's currently defined, we will remove the most fattening carbohydrates from the diet and some portion of total carbohydrates as well. And if we lose fat, this will almost assuredly be the reason why. (This is the opposite of what happens, by the way, when food producers make low-fat products. They remove a little of the fat and its calories, but then replace it with carbohydrates. In the case of low-fat yogurt, for instance, they replace much of the fat removed with high-fructose corn syrup. We think we're eating a heart-healthy, low-fat snack that will lead to weight loss. Instead, we get fatter because of the added carbohydrates and fructose.)

The same is likely to be true for those who swear they lost their excess pounds by taking up regular exercise. Rare are the people who begin running or swimming or doing aerobics five times a week to slim down but don't make any changes in what they eat. Rather, they cut down their beer and soda consumption, reduce

---

*This is something that even researchers who run clinical trials testing the effectiveness of different diets rarely recognize. Imagine we want to cut our daily calories from 2,500 to 1,500, hoping to lose 2 pounds of fat a week. And imagine that the nutrient content of our current diet is what the authorities consider ideal—20 percent protein, 30 percent fat, and 50 percent carbohydrates. That's 500 calories of protein, 750 calories of fat, and 1,250 of carbohydrates. If we keep the same balance of nutrients but eat only 1,500 calories a day, that's 300 calories of protein, 450 calories of fat, and 750 calories of carbohydrates. We've now cut protein calories by 200, fat calories by 300, and carbohydrate calories by 500. If we try to eat even less fat—say, only 25 percent of calories, significantly less than most of us will tolerate—we'll now be eating 300 calories of protein, 375 calories of fat, and 825 of carbohydrates. We've cut our fat calories by 375 a day, but we're still cutting carbohydrates by 425. And if we increase the amount of protein we eat, we'll eat still fewer carbohydrates to compensate.

their sweets, and maybe even try to replace starches with green vegetables.

When calorie-restricted diets fail, as they typically do (and the same can be said of exercise programs), the reason is that they restrict something other than the foods that make us fat. They restrict fat and protein, which have no long-term effect on insulin and fat deposition but are required for energy and for the rebuilding of cells and tissues. They starve the entire body of nutrients and energy, or semi-starve it, rather than targeting the fat tissue specifically. Any weight that might be lost can be maintained only as long as the dieter can withstand the semi-starvation, and even then the fat cells will be working to recoup the fat they're losing, just as the muscle cells are trying to obtain protein to rebuild and maintain their function, and the total amount of energy the dieter expends will be reduced to compensate.

What Adiposity 101 ultimately teaches us is that weight-loss regimens succeed when they get rid of the fattening carbohydrates in the diet; they fail when they don't. What the regimen must do, in essence, is reregulate fat tissue so that it releases the calories it has accumulated to excess. Any changes the dieter makes that don't work toward that goal (reducing the fat and protein consumed, in particular) will starve the body in other ways (of energy, and of protein needed to rebuild muscle), and the resultant hunger will lead to failure.

16

A Historical Digression
on the Fattening Carbohydrate

"Oh Heavens!" all you readers of both sexes will cry out, "oh Heavens above! But what a wretch the Professor is! Here in a single word he forbids us everything we most love, those little white rolls . . . and those cookies . . . and a hundred other things made with flour and butter, with flour and sugar, with flour and sugar and eggs! He doesn't even leave us potatoes, or macaroni! Who would have thought this of a lover of good food who seemed so pleasant?"

"What's this I hear?" I exclaim, putting on my severest face, which I do perhaps once a year. "Very well then; eat! Get fat! Become ugly, and thick, and asthmatic, and finally die in your own melted grease: I shall be there to watch it."

Jean Anthelme Brillat-Savarin, 1825

Jean Anthelme Brillat-Savarin was born in 1755. He became first a lawyer and then a politician. His passion, though, was always food and drink, or what he called the "pleasures of the table." He began writing down his thoughts on the subject in the 1790s; Brillat-Savarin published them in a book, *The Physiology of Taste*, in December 1825. He died of pneumonia two months later, but *The Physiology of Taste* has remained in print ever since. "Tell me what you eat," Brillat-Savarin memorably wrote, "and I shall tell you what you are."

Among the thirty chapters, or "meditations," in *The Physiology of Taste*, Brillat-Savarin included two on obesity—one on cause and one on prevention. Over the course of thirty years, he wrote, he had held more than five hundred conversations with dinner companions who were "threatened or afflicted with obesity," one "fat man" after another, declaring their devotion to bread, rice, pasta, and potatoes. This led Brillat-Savarin to conclude that the roots of obesity were obvious. The first was a natural predisposition to fatten. "Some people," he wrote, "in whom the digestive forces manufacture, all things being equal, a greater supply of fat are, as it were, destined to be obese." The second was "the starches and flours which man uses as the base of his daily nourishment," and he added that "starch produces this effect more quickly and surely when it is used with sugar."

This, of course, made the cure obvious as well. "An anti-fat diet," Brillat-Savarin wrote, "is based on the commonest and most active cause of obesity, since, as it has already been clearly shown, it is only because of grains and starches that fatty congestion can occur, as much in man as in the animals. . . . It can be deduced, as an exact consequence, that a more or less rigid abstinence from everything that is starchy or floury will lead to the lessening of weight."

As I've suggested before, repeating myself on the subject of repetitiousness, very little that I've said so far is new. That includes the idea that carbohydrates cause obesity and that abstinence from starches, flour, and sugars is the obvious method of cure and prevention. What Brillat-Savarin wrote in 1825 has been repeated and reinvented numerous times since. Up through the 1960s, it was the conventional wisdom, what our parents or our grandparents instinctively believed to be true. Then calories-in/calories-out took hold, and the diet that Brillat-Savarin recommended in 1825 and others like it were portrayed by the health authorities as faddish and dangerous—"bizarre concepts of nutrition and dieting," as the American Medical Association described them back in 1973.

By taking this approach, the authorities successfully managed to keep many from trying the diets and certainly succeeded in preventing physicians from recommending them or supporting their use. As Dean Ornish, a diet doctor who became famous for a diet of the opposite nutritional composition (very low in fat and *high* in carbohydrates), has been fond of saying in precisely this context, we can lose weight by using any number of things that aren't good for us—cigarettes and cocaine, for instance—but that doesn't mean any of us should do so.

This is another of the mystifying trends in the past century of diet and nutrition. The notion of the fattening carbohydrate has indeed been around for most of the last two hundred years. Consider, for instance, two novels published nearly a century apart. In Tolstoy's *Anna Karenina*, written in the mid-1870s, Anna's lover, Count Vronsky, abstains from carbohydrates in preparation for the climactic horse race. "On the day of the races at Krasnoe Selo," Tolstoy wrote, "Vronsky had come earlier than usual to eat beefsteak in the officers' mess of the regiment. He had no need to be in strict training, as he had very quickly been brought down to the required weight of one hundred and sixty pounds, but still he had to avoid gaining weight, and he avoided starchy foods and desserts." In 1964, Saul Bellow's Herzog, in the novel by that name, denies himself a candy bar with identical logic, although in Herzog's case, "thinking of the money he had spent on new clothes which would not fit if he ate carbohydrates."

This is what doctors believed and told their obese patients. When physicians stopped believing it, a process that began in the 1960s and concluded in the late 1970s, it happened to coincide with the beginning of the current epidemics of obesity and diabetes. Considering that our physicians have mostly bought into the idea that avoiding carbohydrates as a means of weight loss is a bizarre concept of nutrition, I'd like to review the full history of the idea, so that we can all understand where it comes from and where it went.

A Historical Digression on the Fattening Carbohydrate

. . .

Until the early years of the twentieth century, physicians typically considered obesity a disease, and a virtually incurable one, against which, as with cancer, it was reasonable to try anything. Inducing patients to eat less and/or exercise more was just one of many treatments that might be considered.

In the 1869 edition of *The Practice of Medicine*, the British physician Thomas Tanner published a lengthy list of "ridiculous" treatments that doctors had prescribed for obesity over the years. These included everything from the surreal—"bleeding from the jugular," for instance, and "leeches to the anus"—to elements of today's conventional wisdom, such as eating "very light meals of substances that can be easily digested" and devoting "many hours daily to walking or riding." "All these plans," wrote Tanner, "however perseveringly carried out, fail to accomplish the object desired; and the same must be said of simple sobriety in eating and drinking." (Tanner did believe, however, that abstinence from carbohydrates was one method, perhaps the only one, that worked. "Farinaceous [starchy] and vegetable foods are fattening, and saccharine matters [i.e., sweets] are especially so," he wrote.)

By that time, a French physician and retired military surgeon named Jean-François Dancel had come to the same conclusions as his countryman Brillat-Savarin. Dancel presented his thoughts on obesity in 1844 to the French Academy of Sciences and then published a book, *Obesity, or Excessive Corpulence: The Various Causes and the Rational Means of a Cure*, which was translated into English in 1864. Dancel claimed that he could cure obesity "without a single exception" if he could induce his patients to live "chiefly upon meat," and partake "only of a small quantity of other food."

Dancel argued that physicians of his era believed obesity to be incurable because the diets they prescribed to cure it were precisely those that happened to cause it (an argument implicit in this book, of course, as well). "Medical authors assert that food has a most important bearing in the production of corpulence," he wrote. "They forbid the use of meat, and recommend watery vegetables, such as spinach, sorrel, salad, fruit, &c., and for beverage water; and at the same time they direct the patient to eat as little as possible. I lay it down as an axiom, in opposition to the received opinion of centuries, that very substantial diet, such as meat, does not develop fat and that nothing is more capable of producing the latter than aqueous vegetables and water."

Dancel based his faith in a chiefly meat diet on the work of the German chemist Justus Liebig, who was correctly arguing at the time that fat is formed in animals not from protein but from the ingestion of fats, starches, and sugars. "All food which is not flesh—all food rich in carbon and hydrogen [i.e., carbohydrates]—must have a tendency to produce fat," wrote Dancel. "Upon these principles only can any rational treatment for the cure of obesity satisfactorily rest." Dancel also noted, as Brillat-Savarin had and others would, that carnivorous animals are never fat, whereas herbivores, living exclusively on plants, often are: "The hippopotamus, for example," wrote Dancel, "so uncouth in form from its immense amount of fat, feeds wholly upon vegetable matter—rice, millet, sugarcane, &c."

The diet was then reinvented by William Harvey, a British doctor, after visiting Paris in 1856 and watching the legendary Claude Bernard lecture on diabetes. As Harvey later told it, Bernard described how the liver secretes glucose, the same carbohydrate that can be found in sugar and starch, and it's the level of this glucose in the blood that is abnormally elevated in diabetics. This led Harvey to consider what was then a well-known fact, that a diet absent any sugar and starches would curb the secretion of sugar in the urine of a diabetic. He then speculated that the same diet might work as a weight-loss diet as well.

"Knowing too that a saccharine [sweet] and farinaceous [starchy] diet is used to fatten certain animals," Harvey wrote, "and that in diabetes the whole of the fat of the body rapidly disappears, it occurred to me that excessive obesity might be allied to diabetes as to its cause, although widely diverse in its development; and that if a purely animal diet were useful in the latter disease, a combination of animal food with such vegetable diet as contained neither sugar nor starch, might serve to arrest the undue formation of fat."

In August 1862, Harvey prescribed his diet for an obese London undertaker named William Banting (whom I introduced briefly in an earlier chapter, talking about his rowing experiences). By the following May, Banting had lost thirty-five pounds—he eventually lost fifty—prompting him to publish a sixteen-page *Letter on Corpulence* that described his previous weight-loss attempts, all futile, and his effortless success when living on meat, fish, game, and no more than a few ounces of fruit or stale toast a day. (Banting's diet did include a considerable amount of alcohol—four or five glasses of wine each day, a cordial every morning, and an evening tumbler of gin, whisky, or brandy.)

"Bread, butter, milk, sugar, beer, and potatoes," Banting wrote, "had been the main (and, I thought, innocent) elements of my subsistence, or at all events they had for many years been adopted freely. These, said my excellent adviser, contain starch and saccharine matter, tending to create fat, and should be avoided altogether. At the first blush it seemed to me that I had little left to live upon, but my kind friend soon showed me there was ample. I was only too happy to give the plan a fair trial, and, within a very few days, found immense benefit from it."

Banting's *Letter on Corpulence* became an instant best-seller and was translated widely. By the autumn of 1864, even the emperor of France was "trying the Banting system and is said to have already profited greatly thereby." Banting credited Harvey for the diet, but it was Banting's name that entered the English language (and the Swedish) as a verb meaning "to diet," and it was Banting who took the heat from the medical community. "We advise Mr Banting, and everyone of his kind, not to meddle with medical literature again, but be content to mind his own business," wrote *The Lancet*, a British medical journal.

Still, when the Congress of Internal Medicine met in Berlin in 1886 and held a session on popular diets, Banting's diet was considered one of three that could now reliably be used to reduce obese patients. The other two were minor variations developed by renowned German physicians—one prescribed even more fat, and the other (based on Dancel's work) less fluid, leaner meat, and exercise. Both allowed unlimited meat consumption but prohibited starches and sweets almost entirely.

When Hilde Bruch recounted this history in 1957, she noted that the treatment of obesity hadn't changed much in the intervening decades. "The great progress in dietary control of obesity was the recognition that meat, 'the strong food,' was not fat producing," she wrote; "but that it was innocent foodstuffs, such as bread and sweets, which lead to obesity."

It's hard to imagine today how widely held was this notion, considering the attempts by the authorities in the last forty years to tar it as a recurring fad. Let me list some examples of the advice on weight loss taken from the medical literature up through the 1960s.

In the 1901 edition of *The Principles and Practice of Medicine*, William Osler, considered the father of modern medicine in North America, advises obese women to "avoid taking too much food, and particularly to reduce the starches and sugars."

In 1907, James French, in *A Text-book of the Practice of Medicine* says, "The overappropriation of nourishment seen in obesity is derived in part from the fat ingested with the food, but more particularly from the carbohydrates."

In 1925, H. Gardiner-Hill of London's St. Thomas's Hospital Medical School describes his carbohydrate-restricted diet in *The Lancet*: "All forms of bread contain a large proportion of carbohydrate, varying from 45–65 percent, and the percentage in toast may be as high as 60. It should thus be condemned."

Between 1943 and 1952, physicians from the Stanford University School of Medicine, Harvard Medical School, Children's Memorial Hospital in Chicago, and from Cornell Medical School and New York Hospital independently published their diets for treating obese patients. All four are effectively identical. Here are the "General Rules" of the Chicago version:

1. Do not use sugar, honey, syrup, jam, jelly or candy.
2. Do not use fruits canned with sugar.
3. Do not use cake, cookies, pie, puddings, ice cream or ices.
4. Do not use foods which have cornstarch or flour added such as gravy or cream sauce.
5. Do not use potatoes (sweet or Irish), macaroni, spaghetti, noodles, dried beans or peas.
6. Do not use fried foods prepared with butter, lard, oil or butter substitutes.
7. Do not use drinks such as Coca-Cola, ginger ale, pop or root beer.
8. Do not use any foods not allowed on the diet and only as much as the diet allows.

And here's the obesity diet published in the 1951 textbook *The Practice of Endocrinology*, coedited by seven prominent British physicians led by Raymond Greene, probably the most influential twentieth-century British endocrinologist (and brother of the novelist Graham Greene):

Foods to be avoided:

1. Bread, and everything else made with flour . . .
2. Cereals, including breakfast cereals and milk puddings
3. Potatoes and all other white root vegetables
4. Foods containing much sugar
5. All sweets . . .

You can eat as much as you like of the following foods:

1. Meat, fish, birds
2. All green vegetables
3. Eggs, dried or fresh
4. Cheese
5. Fruit, if unsweetened or sweetened with saccharin, except bananas and grapes

Welcome to what was once the conventional wisdom. It was so ingrained that when the U.S. Navy was steaming west across the Pacific in the endgame of World War II, the official *U.S. Forces' Guide* warned soldiers that they might have "trouble with girth control" in the Caroline Islands, an archipelago northeast of New Guinea, because "the basic food the natives eat is starchy vegetables—breadfruit, taro, yams, sweet potatoes, and arrowroot."

In 1946, when the very first edition of Dr. Spock's child-rearing bible, *Baby and Child Care*, was published, it counseled, "The amount of plain, starchy foods (cereals, breads, potatoes) taken is what determines, in the case of most people, how much [weight] they gain or lose." And that sentence remained in every edition—five more, constituting in total some fifty million copies—for the next fifty years.

In 1963, when Sir Stanley Davidson and Reginald Passmore published *Human Nutrition and Dietetics*, considered the definitive source of dietary wisdom for a generation of British medical practitioners, they wrote, "All popular 'slimming regimes' involve a restriction in dietary carbohydrate," and advised, "The intake of foods rich in carbohydrate should be drastically reduced since over-indulgence in such foods is the most common cause of obesity." The same year, Passmore co-authored an article in the *British Journal of Nutrition* that began with this declaration: "Every woman knows that carbohydrate is fattening: this is a piece of common knowledge, which few nutritionists would dispute."

A Historical Digression on the Fattening Carbohydrate

. . .

By this time, physicians had taken to testing the effectiveness of diets that restricted carbohydrates, and they began reporting on these tests and their own clinical experience. (The first was in 1936 by Per Hanssen, a physician at Steno Memorial Hospital in Copenhagen.) The results were unambiguous: the diets seemed to induce significant weight loss without requiring that the patients go hungry.

The pioneering studies were done at the DuPont Company in Delaware in the late 1940s. "We had urged our overweight employees to cut down on the size of the portions they ate, to count their calories, to limit the amounts of fats and carbohydrates in their meals, to get more exercise," explained George Gehrmann, head of the company's industrial-medicine division. "None of those things had worked." So Gehrmann had his colleague Alfred Pennington look into the problem, and Pennington prescribed a mostly meat diet to twenty overweight employees. They lost an average of two pounds a week, rarely eating fewer than twenty-four hundred calories a day and averaging three thousand calories, or twice that typically prescribed in the semi-starvation diets that we're still being told to follow today. "Notable was a lack of hunger between meals," Pennington wrote, "increased physical energy and sense of well being." The DuPont subjects were allowed no more than eighty calories of carbohydrates per meal. "In a few cases," Pennington reported, "even this much carbohydrate prevented weight loss, though an [unrestricted] intake of protein and fat, more exclusively, was successful."

Pennington's conclusions were then confirmed in the 1950s by Margaret Ohlson, head of the nutrition department at Michigan State University, and by her student Charlotte Young, working at Cornell University. When overweight students were put on conventional semi-starvation diets, Ohlson reported, they lost little weight and "reported a lack of 'pep' throughout . . . [and] they were discouraged because they were always conscious of being hungry." When they ate only a few hundred carbohydrate calories a day but plenty of protein and fat, they lost an average of three pounds per week and "reported a feeling of well-being and satisfaction. Hunger between meals was not a problem."

The reports continued into the 1970s. Some physicians prescribed carbohydrate restriction with a limit to how much fat and protein could be eaten—allowing anywhere from six hundred total calories a day to twenty-one hundred—and some prescribed the diet as an "eat as much as you like diet," which means as much meat, fowl, and fish as desired, as much protein and fat, but still very few carbohydrates. Some physicians allowed virtually no carbohydrates, not even green vegetables. Some allowed as much as four hundred calories' worth. These studies were carried out at hospitals and universities in the United States, the United Kingdom, Canada, Cuba, France, Germany, Sweden, and Switzerland. The diets were prescribed for obese adults and children, for men and women, and the results were invariably the same. The dieters lost weight with little effort and felt little or no hunger while doing so.

By the mid-1960s, when physicians began holding regular conferences dedicated to obesity, the conferences invariably included a single talk on dietary therapy, and that talk invariably was on the unique effectiveness of carbohydrate-restricted diets.* Five of these conferences were held in the United States and Europe between 1967 and 1974. The largest was at the National Institutes of Health in Bethesda, Maryland, in October 1973. The talk on dietary treatment was given by Charlotte Young of Cornell.

Young reviewed the hundred-year history of the fattening carbohydrate, including Pennington's work at Dupont and Ohlson's

---

* These conferences did not include a discussion of calorie-restricted diets for obesity, because these physicians already knew that calorie-restricted diets failed in virtually all cases. Occasionally, however, they did include a discussion of the efficacy of fasting entirely, which succeeded but only as long as the patients continued fasting.

at Michigan State. She talked about her own work, putting obese young men on diets of eighteen hundred calories. These diets all included the same amount of protein, but some had virtually no carbohydrates and a lot of fat; some had a few hundred calories of carbohydrates and not quite so much fat. "Weight loss, fat loss, and percent weight loss as fat appeared to be inversely related to the level of carbohydrate in the diets," Young reported. In other words, the fewer carbohydrates these men ate and the more fat, the more weight they lost and the more body fat they lost—exactly what Adiposity 101 would have predicted. What's more, all of these carbohydrate-restricted diets, Young said, "gave excellent clinical results as measured by freedom from hunger, allaying of excessive fatigue, satisfactory weight loss, suitability for long term weight reduction and subsequent weight control."

Now, you might think that, given these results, confirmed in studies around the world, and given the science of fat metabolism— Adiposity 101—which had by then been worked out in detail, the medical community and the public health authorities might have had an epiphany. Perhaps they might have launched a campaign to convince individuals who gain weight easily that they should avoid, at the very least, the most fattening of carbohydrate-rich foods—the refined, easily digestible carbohydrates and sugars. But this obviously isn't what happened.

By the 1960s, obesity had come to be perceived as an eating disorder, and so the actual science of fat regulation, as I said previously, wasn't considered relevant (as it still isn't). Adiposity 101 was discussed in the physiology, endocrinology, and biochemistry journals, but rarely crossed over into the medical journals or the literature on obesity itself. When it did, as in a lengthy article in *The Journal of the American Medical Association* in 1963, it was ignored. Few doctors were willing to accept a cure for obesity predicated on the notion that fat people can eat large portions of any food, let alone as much as they want. This simply ran contrary to what had now come to be accepted as the obvious reason why fat people get fat to begin with, that they eat too much.

But there was another problem as well. Health officials had come to believe that dietary fat causes heart disease, and that carbohydrates are what these authorities would come to call "heart-healthy." This is why the famous Food Guide Pyramid of the U.S. Department of Agriculture would later put fats and oils at the top, to be "used sparingly"; meat was near the top because meat (like fish and fowl to a lesser extent) has considerable fat in it—even lean meat—and fat-free carbohydrates—or fattening carbohydrates, as they used to be known—were at the bottom, the staples of a supposedly healthy diet.

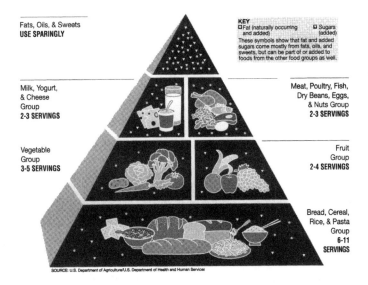

This belief in the carbohydrate as "heart-healthy" started in the 1960s and it couldn't be reconciled with the idea that carbohydrates make us fat. After all, if dietary fat causes heart attacks, then a diet that replaces carbohydrates with more fatty foods threatens to kill us, even if it slims us down in the process. As a result, doctors and nutritionists started attacking carbohydrate-restricted diets, because they bought into an idea about heart disease that was barely even tested at the time and would fail to be confirmed once it was (as I will soon discuss). They believed it, though, because people they respected believed it, and those people believed it because, well, other people they respected believed it.

A particularly glaring example comes from *The New York Times* in 1965, the same year the American Physiological Society published an eight-hundred-page *Handbook of Physiology* dedicated to the science of fat metabolism, a subject I addressed in the previous chapter, and concluding, effectively, that "carbohydrate is driving insulin is driving fat."

The *Times* article, "New Diet Decried by Nutritionists: Dangers Are Seen in Low Carbohydrate Intake," quoted Harvard's Jean Mayer as claiming that to prescribe carbohydrate-restricted diets to the public was "the equivalent of mass murder."

Mass murder.

Mayer's logic? Well, first, as the *Times* explained, "It is a medical fact that no dieter can lose weight unless he cuts down on excess calories, either by taking in fewer of them, or by burning them up." We now know that this is not a medical fact, but the nutritionists didn't in 1965, and most of them still don't. Second, because these diets restrict carbohydrates, they compensate by allowing more fat. It's the high-fat nature of the diets, the *Times* explained, that prompted Mayer to make the mass murder accusation.

This is how such diets have been treated ever since. The belief that dietary fat causes heart disease—saturated fat, particularly—led directly to the idea that carbohydrates prevent it. By the early 1980s, Jane Brody of the *Times*, the single most influential journalist on the nutrition beat for the last forty years, was telling us "we need to eat more carbohydrates" and advocating starches and bread as diet foods. "Not only is eating pasta at the height of fashion," she wrote, "it can help you lose weight." In 1983, when British authorities compiled their "Proposals for Nutritional Guidelines for Health Education in Britain," they had to explain that "the previous nutritional advice in the UK to limit the intake of all carbohydrates as a means of weight control now runs counter to current thinking."

This logic may have reached the pinnacle of absurdity in 1995 (at least I hope it did), when the American Heart Association published a pamphlet suggesting that we can eat virtually anything with impunity—even candy and sugar—as long as it's low in fat: "To control the amount and kind of fat, saturated fatty acids and dietary cholesterol you eat," the AHA counseled, "choose snacks from other food groups such as . . . low-fat cookies, low-fat crackers . . . unsalted pretzels, hard candy, gum drops, sugar, syrup, honey, jam, jelly, marmalade (as spreads)."

This advice and the shunning of low-carbohydrate weight-loss diets might make sense if dietary fat did indeed cause heart disease, as we've been hearing now for fifty years. But there has always been copious evidence suggesting that this obsession with dietary fat is misdirected—another case of the health authorities fooling first themselves, and then the rest of us, because they thought they knew the truth about a subject in advance of actually doing any meaningful research. In the next chapter, I'll discuss what the history of our species has to say about whether a diet that prohibits *only* the fattening carbohydrates—starches, anything made from flour, sugars—is healthy or not, even if it means eating significant fat and meat instead. In the chapter that follows, I'll discuss what the latest medical research says about the nature of a healthy diet.

17

Meat or Plants?

In 1919, a New York cardiologist named Blake Donaldson began prescribing mostly meat diets to his obese and overweight patients—"fat cardiacs," he called them, because even ninety years ago these men were obviously prime candidates for a heart attack. As Donaldson told it, he had visited the local Museum of Natural History and asked the resident anthropologists what our prehistoric ancestors ate, and they told him "the fattest meat they could kill," with some minimal roots and berries for variety. So Donaldson decided that fatty meat should be "the essential part of any reducing diet," and this is what he prescribed to his patients: half a pound three times a day, with a small portion of fruit or potato to substitute for the berries and roots. Donaldson continued with this prescription until he retired forty years later, successfully treating (or so he claimed) seventeen thousand patients for their weight problems.*

Donaldson may or may not have been ahead of his time, but the argument that we should eat what we evolved to eat has remained forceful ever since. The idea is that the longer a particular type of food has been part of the human diet, the more bene-

---

*It was Donaldson's diet that led Alfred Pennington to treat DuPont executives with mostly meat diets in the late 1940s, and Pennington's work that led Herman Taller, a New York obstetrician, to write *Calories Don't Count*, which became one of the most controversial diet books ever written and, in the process, shaped much of the debate, still ongoing obviously, about carbohydrates and carbohydrate-restricted diets.

ficial and less harmful it probably is—the better adapted we become to that food. And if some food is new to human diets, or new in large quantities, it's likely that we haven't yet had time to adapt, and so it's doing us harm.

This logic is implicit in virtually all public-health recommendations about chronic-disease prevention. It was set forth explicitly in the 1980s by Geoffrey Rose, a British epidemiologist, in a pair of articles—"Strategy of Prevention" and "Sick Individuals and Sick Populations"—that would take their place among the most influential articles in public health. The only measures that public-health officials can recommend as means of preventing chronic disease, Rose said, are those that remove "unnatural factors" and restore " 'biological normality'—that is . . . the conditions to which presumably we are genetically adapted. . . . Such normalizing measures may be presumed to be safe, and therefore we should be prepared to advocate them on the basis of a reasonable presumption of benefit."

The obvious question is, what are the "conditions to which presumably we are genetically adapted"? As it turns out, what Donaldson assumed in 1919 is still the conventional wisdom today: our genes were effectively shaped by the two and a half million years during which our ancestors lived as hunters and gatherers prior to the introduction of agriculture twelve thousand years ago. This is a period of time known as the Paleolithic era or, less technically, as the Stone Age, because it begins with the development of the first stone tools. It constitutes more than 99.5 percent of human history—more than a hundred thousand generations of humanity living as hunter-gatherers, compared with the six hundred succeeding generations of farmers or the ten generations that have lived in the industrial age.

It's not controversial to say that the agricultural period—the last .5 percent of the history of our species—has had little significant effect on our genetic makeup. What is significant is what we ate during the two and a half million years that preceded agriculture—the Paleolithic era. The question can never be answered definitively, because this era, after all, preceded human record-keeping. The best we can do is what nutritional anthropologists began doing in the mid-1980s—use modern-day hunter-gatherer societies as surrogates for our Stone Age ancestors.

In 2000, researchers from the United States and Australia published an analysis of the diets of 229 hunter-gatherer populations that survived deep enough into the twentieth century to have their diets assessed by anthropologists.* This analysis is still considered the most comprehensive ever done on the subject of modern-day hunter-gatherer diets and so, by implication, about the nature of the diets, as Rose would have said, "to which presumably we are genetically adapted." Four of its conclusions are relevant to our question of whether a diet that makes us lean— one absent fattening carbohydrates—can be a healthy diet.

First, "whenever and wherever it was ecologically possible," hunter-gatherers consumed "high amounts" of animal food. In fact, one in every five of these 229 populations subsisted almost entirely by hunting or fishing. These populations got more than 85 percent of their calories from meat or fish; some got 100 percent. This alone tells us that it's possible to survive, if not thrive, on diets completely lacking fruits, vegetables, and grains. Only 14 percent of these hunter-gatherer populations got more than half their calories from plant foods. Not a single one of these populations was exclusively vegetarian. When averaged all together, these hunter-gatherer populations consumed about two-thirds of their total calories from animal foods and one third from plants.

The second lesson is about the fat-and-protein content of these diets. For the past fifty years, we've been told to eat low-fat diets—as the USDA Food Guide Pyramid counsels—and we certainly have made an attempt to do so. On average, we get 15 percent of our calories from protein, 33 percent from fat, and the remainder (more than 50 percent) from carbohydrates. But these modern hunter-gatherers ate quite differently, and so in all proba-

*By Loren Cordain et al.; see Sources.

bility did our Paleolithic ancestors. Their diets were high to very high in protein compared with today (19 to 35 percent of calories), and high to very high in fat (28 to 58 percent of calories). And some of these populations consumed as much as 80 percent of their calories from fat, as the Inuits did, for instance, before they traded with Europeans and added sugar and flour to their diets.

Hunter-gatherers, as these researchers explained, preferentially ate the fattest animals they could hunt; they preferentially ate the fattest parts of the animal, including organs, tongue, and bone marrow, and they would eat "virtually all" of the fat on the animal. In other words, they preferred fatty meat and organs to the kind of lean muscle meat that we now buy at the supermarket or order in restaurants.*

Third, the diets were low in carbohydrates "by normal Western standards"—*averaging* from 22 to 40 percent of energy. One obvious reason for this is that these hunter-gatherers preferred meat if they could get it. Another is that wild plant foods have "relatively low carbohydrate content" compared with the floury foods and starches we eat today. All of the plant foods that these populations gathered (seeds, nuts, roots, tubers, bulbs, "miscellaneous plant parts," and fruits) would have what nutritionists today call a low glycemic index: they would be very slow to raise blood sugar, which would dictate an equally slow and measured insulin response. Not only would these hunter-gatherers eat relatively few carbohydrates, but what digestible carbohydrates they did eat would be bound up tightly with indigestible fiber, making the great majority of these plant foods very difficult and slow to digest. (One argument seriously discussed today for the invention of cooking is that it was first used to render tubers and other plant foods edible. Only later was it used to roast meat.) Simply put, they wouldn't be fattening.

The one thing we can say for sure, as this analysis did, is that

---

*The same behavior is typical of carnivores. Lions, for instance, will eat the fat organ meat of their kills and leave the "lean muscle meat" for scavengers.

this hunter-gatherer diet is a far cry from the recommended diet today, which includes carbohydrate-rich, easily digestible starches and grains—including corn, potatoes, rice, wheat, and beans. In fact, all the carbohydrate-rich foods that Adiposity 101 (and anecdotal evidence, at least until the 1960s) tells us are fattening are very new additions to human diets. Indeed, many of these foods have been available for only the past few hundred years—the last thousandth of a percent of our two and a half million years on the planet. Corn and potatoes originated as New World vegetables and spread to Europe and then Asia only after Columbus; the machine refining of flour and sugar dates only to the late nineteenth century. Just two hundred years ago, we ate less than a fifth of the sugar we eat today.

Even the fruits we eat today are vastly different from the wild varieties consumed by hunter-gatherers, whether the modern versions or the Paleolithic ones. And they're now available year-round, rather than for only a few months of the year—late summer and fall in temperate climates. Although nutritionists today consider copious fruit a necessary part of a healthy diet, and it has become popular to suggest that one problem with Western diets is the relative absence of fruit, it's worth remembering that we've been cultivating fruit trees for only the past few thousand years, and that the kinds of fruit we eat today—Fuji apples, Bartlett pears, navel oranges—have been bred to be far juicier and sweeter than the wild varieties and so, in effect, to be far more fattening.

The essential point, as this 2000 analysis noted, is that the modern foods that today constitute more than 60 percent of all calories in the typical Western diet—including cereal grains, dairy products, beverages, vegetable oils and dressings, and sugar and candy—"would have contributed virtually none of the energy in the typical hunter-gatherer diet." If we believe that our genetic makeup has a say in what constitutes a healthy diet, then the likely reason that easily digestible starches, refined carbohydrates (flour and white rice), and sugars are fattening is that we didn't evolve to eat them and certainly not in the quantities in which we eat them today. That a diet would be healthier without them seems manifestly obvious. As for meat, fish, and fowl, for protein and fat, these would be the staples of a healthy diet, as they apparently were for our ancestors for two and a half million years.

If we turn this evolutionary argument on its head, we come to the experience of isolated populations that go from eating their traditional diets to incorporating the kinds of foods that we eat daily in modern Westernized societies. Public-health experts call this a "nutrition transition," and it's invariably accompanied by a disease transition as well—the appearance of a collection of chronic diseases that are now known as Western diseases for just this reason. These diseases include obesity, diabetes, heart disease, hypertension and stroke, cancer, Alzheimer's disease and other dementias, cavities, periodontal disease, appendicitis, ulcers, diverticulitis, gallstones, hemorrhoids, varicose veins, and constipation. These diseases and conditions are common in societies that eat Western diets and live modern lifestyles, and they're uncommon, if not nonexistent, in societies that don't. And when those traditional societies take up Western diets and lifestyles—through either trade or emigration (voluntary or forced, as in the slave trade)—these diseases will appear shortly after.

This association of chronic diseases with modern diets and lifestyle was first noted in the mid-nineteenth century, when a French physician named Stanislas Tanchou pointed out that "cancer, like insanity, seems to increase with the progress of civilization." Now, as Michael Pollan points out, it's one of the indisputable facts of diet and health. Eat Western diets, get Western diseases—notably obesity, diabetes, heart disease, and cancer.*

---

*In 1997, John Higginson, the founding director of the World Health Organization's International Agency for Cancer Research, described as a "cultural

This is one of the primary reasons why public-health experts believe that there are dietary and lifestyle causes for all these diseases, even cancer—that they're not just the result of bad luck or bad genes.

To get a feel for the kind of modern evidence supporting this idea, consider breast cancer. In Japan, this disease is relatively rare, certainly not the scourge it is for American women. But when Japanese women emigrate to the United States, it takes only two generations for their descendants to experience the same breast-cancer rates as any other local ethnic group. This tells us that something about the American lifestyle or diet is causing breast cancer. The question is what. We could say that something about the Japanese diet or lifestyle protects against breast cancer, but similar trends have been seen among the Inuits, in whom breast cancer was virtually nonexistent until the 1960s; the Pima; and a host of other populations as well. In all these populations, the frequency of breast cancer is low to very low on traditional diets, and it goes up significantly, if not dramatically, when they become Westernized.

There's little controversy about this. It appears again and again in virtually all the studies of Western diseases. Colon cancer is ten times more common in rural Connecticut than in Nigeria. Alzheimer's disease is far more common among Japanese Americans than among Japanese living in Japan; it's twice as common among African Americans as among rural Africans. Pick a disease from the list of Western diseases, and a pair of locations—one urban, say, and one rural, or one Westernized and one not—compare people in the same age groups, and the disease will be more

---

shock" the experience of training to be a doctor in Europe or North America and then going off to work in one of these non-Westernized societies, as he had done in South Africa a half-century earlier. The physicians discover, he wrote, "that the patterns and pathogenesis of disease . . . were very different from what they had been accustomed to elsewhere. Moreover, such differences were not confined to the communicable diseases as anticipated, but also the chronic illness such as cancer and heart disease."

common in the urban and Westernized locations and less common outside them.

Mainstream nutritionists and public-health authorities have responded to these observations by indicting all aspects of what they believe is the prevailing modern Western diet and lifestyle. They define the Western diet as copious meat, processed food, sugar, and total calories, with few vegetables, fruits, or whole grains. They define the Western lifestyle as sedentary. If we stay away from meat, they tell us, avoid processed foods and sugars, eat less or at least not too much, eat mostly plants and more fruit, and exercise, we'll prevent these diseases and live longer.

The problem with this approach is the basic assumption that everything about the Western diet is bad, and so they can incriminate all of it and feel they've done their job. (This approach reminds me of the story of the thirteenth-century Inquisitors who set out to sack a city of heretics—Béziers, in southwestern France—only to realize that they couldn't tell the heretics from the good Catholics. "Kill them all," they were instructed, "and let God sort them out," and so they did.) What if only some aspects of the Western diet are deleterious to our health and the rest are perfectly benign or even beneficial? After all, lung cancer is also a Western disease, but we don't blame that on the Western diet and sedentary lives, only on cigarettes. And the reason we know cigarettes are responsible is that we know that nonsmokers are relatively free from lung cancer whereas smokers get it frequently.

It's useful (as it is when any crime is committed) to narrow down the list of suspects. First of all, among the non-Westernized populations that have been well studied, quite a few that were exclusively meat eaters, or meat and fish eaters, and so ate no fruits and vegetables at all—the Inuits, again, are an example, as are the Maasai—suffered little or no cancer (or heart disease, diabetes, or obesity). This suggests that meat eating is not a cause of these diseases, and it suggests that copious fruits and vegetables are not necessary to prevent them. In fact, when the disparity in cancer rates between Western and non-Westernized societies was first actively studied a century ago, the idea that meat eating caused cancer, and that isolated populations were protected against it by eating mostly plants, was raised. It was dismissed for the same reason it should be dismissed now: it failed to explain why cancer was prevalent among vegetarian societies—the Hindus in India, for instance, "to whom the fleshpot is an abomination," as one British physician described it in 1899—and rare to absent among the Inuits, Maasai, Native Americans of the Great Plains, and other decidedly carnivorous populations.*

Clearly, as Pollan points out, humans can adapt to a wide range of non-Western diets, from those exclusively animal-based to those mostly, if not exclusively, vegetarian. If all of those populations were relatively free from Western diseases, as they apparently were, the more logical question to ask is what is it that distinguishes Western diets from the diets of all these populations, not just some of them (the ones that eat copious vegetables and fruits, for instance, and little meat). The answer, it turns out, is the same foods that were absent entirely among the hunter-gatherer populations (in which Western diseases were also mostly absent): "cereal grains, dairy products, beverages, vegetable oils and dressings, and sugar and candy."

Researchers who studied this evidence in the 1950s and 1960s—Thomas "Peter" Cleave and George Campbell, co-authors of *Diabetes, Coronary Thrombosis and the Saccharine Disease* (1966), deserve the most credit—made the point that when isolated populations start eating Western foods, sugar and white flour are invariably the first, because these foods could be transported around the world as items of trade without spoiling or

---

*The meat-eating hypothesis "hardly holds good" in regard to Native Americans, as the Columbia University pathologist Isaac Levin noted in 1910. "They consume a great deal of food [rich in nitrogen—i.e., meat], frequently to excess," and yet had virtually no cancer, as Levin himself had confirmed in a survey of physicians from the Office of Indian Affairs working on reservations throughout the American West and Midwest.

being devoured on the way by rodents or insects. The Inuits, for example, living on seals, caribou, and whale meat, begin eating sugar and flour (crackers and bread). Western diseases follow. The agrarian Kikuyu, living in Kenya, start eating sugar and flour, and these diseases appear. South Pacific islanders living on pigs, coconuts, and fish start eating sugar and white flour, and these diseases appear. The Maasai add sugar and flour to their diet or move into the cities and begin eating these foods, and the diseases appear. Even the vegetarian Hindus in India, to whom the fleshpot was an abomination, ate sugar and flour. Doesn't it seem a good idea to consider sugar and flour likely causes of these diseases?

This seems perfectly reasonable to me (and to you, I hope). But it was rejected for the same reason the fattening carbohydrate and carbohydrate-restricted diets were rejected: it clashed with the idea that dietary fat causes heart disease, which had become the preferred hypothesis of nutritionists in the United States. And these nutritionists were simply unaware of the historical and geographical depth of the evidence implicating sugar and flour.

So now we need to revisit the question of whether it's the fat we eat that really causes heart disease. If dietary fat doesn't, we should have a pretty good idea what does. In the next chapter, I'll look at what the latest research shows concerning this question of the dietary causes of heart disease, not to mention diabetes, cancer, and the other diseases of Western diets that we would like to avoid.

18

The Nature of a Healthy Diet

Since carbohydrates make us fat, it follows that the best and perhaps only way to avoid becoming fat is to avoid the carbohydrate-rich foods that are responsible. For those who are already fat, this implies that the best and perhaps only way to become lean again is to do the same. The logic is straightforward. But our doctors believe these diets will do us more harm than good, which makes it a difficult and dangerous proposition to believe otherwise.

Here are the three primary arguments against carbohydrate-restricted diets, the ones that have been made repeatedly since the 1960s:

1) That they're scams because they promise weight loss without having to eat less and/or exercise, thus violating the laws of thermodynamics and the primacy of calories-in/calories-out.

2) That they're unbalanced, because they restrict an entire nutrient category—carbohydrates—and the first law of healthy eating is to eat a balanced diet from all the major food groups.

3) That they're high-fat diets, and particularly high in saturated fat, and will cause heart disease by raising our cholesterol.

Let's take these criticisms one at a time and see how they stand up.

The Con Job Argument

This needs little more discussion. Much of the antagonism toward carbohydrate-restricted diets, from the earliest days, arises from the belief that proponents of these diets are trying to con a gullible public. Eat as much as you want and lose weight? Impossible.

But we know now what happens when we restrict carbohydrates, and why this leads to weight loss and particularly fat loss, independent of the calories we consume from dietary fat and protein. We know that the laws of physics have nothing to do with it.

The Unbalanced Diet Argument

The unbalanced diet argument makes little sense if starches, refined carbohydrates, and sugars do indeed make us fat, because it's hard to argue rationally for anything other than avoiding these carbohydrates to fix the problem. When our doctors counsel us to quit smoking because cigarettes cause lung cancer, emphysema, and heart disease, they don't care if we find life less fulfilling without them. They want us to be healthy, and they assume we'll get over the absence, given time. Since these carbohydrates make us fat—and maybe cause a host of other chronic diseases, as I'll discuss—the same logic holds here.

If you cut back on all calories equally, or preferentially restrict fat calories, as we're often counseled, you'll be eating less fat and protein, which are not fattening, and more of the carbohydrates that are. Not only won't this diet work as well, if it works at all, but hunger will be a constant companion. If you restrict only carbohydrates, you can always eat more protein and fat if you feel the urge, since they have no effect on fat accumulation. As early as 1936, the Danish physician Per Hanssen was pointing out that this was a primary advantage of carbohydrate restriction: if you can lose weight without hunger, aren't you more likely to maintain that way of eating than one that requires indefinite semistarvation?

The argument that a diet that restricts fattening carbohydrates will be lacking in essential nutrients—including vitamins, minerals, amino acids—does not hold up. First, the foods that you would be avoiding are the fattening ones, not leafy green vegetables and salads. This alone should take care of any superficial anxieties about vitamin or mineral deficiencies. Moreover, the fattening carbohydrates that are restricted—starches, refined carbohydrates, and sugars—are virtually absent essential nutrients in any case.*

Even if you believe that weight loss requires cutting calories, these fattening carbohydrates would be the ideal foods to cut for just this reason. If you follow the conventional wisdom and so cut all calories, say, by a third, you're also cutting all essential nutrients by a third. A diet that prohibits sugars, flour, potatoes, and beer, but allows unlimited meat, eggs, and leafy green vegetables, leaves in all the essential nutrients, as the British nutritionist John Yudkin argued in the 1960s and 1970s, and may even increase them, since you can eat more of these particular foods on such a diet, not less.

Ever since the 1960s, when it was first argued that animal products could be bad for our health because they contain saturated fat, nutritionists have typically refrained from pointing out that meat contains all the amino acids necessary for life,† all the

---

*The exceptions are those that are added back in the refining process, such as into "fortified" white bread. Bread manufacturers refine the flour until there's nothing in it of any value except the calories, then add back folic acid and niacin, which is a B vitamin.

†As the late Marvin Harris, a Columbia University nutritional anthropologist, explained, a 175-pound man can get all the protein and amino acids he needs from eating wheat, but to do so he has to "stuff himself" on more than three pounds of it a day. He can get the same level of protein from three-quarters of a pound of meat.

essential fats, and twelve of the thirteen essential vitamins in surprisingly large quantities. It's true nonetheless. Meat is a particularly concentrated source of vitamins A and E, and the entire complex of B vitamins. Vitamins B_{12} and D are found *only* in animal products (although we can get sufficient vitamin D from regular exposure to sunlight).

Vitamin C is the one vitamin that is relatively scarce in animal products. But it appears to be the case, as it certainly is for the B vitamins, that the more fattening carbohydrates we consume, the more of these vitamins we need. We use B vitamins to metabolize glucose in our cells. So, the more carbohydrates we consume, the more glucose we burn (instead of fatty acids), and the more B vitamins we need from our diets.

Vitamin C uses the same mechanism to get into cells (where it's needed) that glucose does, so the higher our blood sugar level, the more glucose enters the cells and the less vitamin C. Insulin also inhibits what's called the uptake of vitamin C by the kidney, which means that when we eat carbohydrates we excrete vitamin C with our urine rather than retaining it, as we should, and using it. Without carbohydrates in the diet, there's every indication that we would get all the vitamin C we ever needed from animal products.

This makes sense from an evolutionary perspective as well, since any human populations that lived far enough from the equator to see lengthy winters would have gone months, if not years, at a time—during ice ages, for instance—without eating anything but what they could hunt. The idea that they required orange juice or fresh vegetables to get their requisite vitamin C every day seems absurd. This would also explain why isolated hunter-gatherer populations that ate virtually no carbohydrates and certainly no green vegetables or fruits still thrived.

Carbohydrates are not required in a healthy human diet. Another way to say this (as proponents of carbohydrate restriction have) is that there is no such thing as an essential carbohydrate. Nutritionists will say that 120 to 130 grams of carbohydrates are required in a healthy diet, but this is because they confuse what the brain and central nervous system will burn for fuel when diets are carbohydrate rich—120 to 130 grams daily—with what we actually have to eat.

If there are no carbohydrates in the diet, the brain and central nervous system will run on molecules called "ketones." These are synthesized in the liver from the fat we eat and from fatty acids, mobilized from the fat tissue because we're not eating carbohydrates and insulin levels are low, and even from some amino acids. With no carbohydrates in the diet, ketones will provide roughly three-quarters of the energy that our brains use. And this is why severely carbohydrate-restricted diets are known as "*keto-genic*" diets. The rest of the energy required will come from glycerol, which is also being released from the fat tissue when the triglycerides are broken down into their component parts, and from glucose synthesized in the liver from the amino acids in protein. Because a diet that doesn't include fattening carbohydrates will still include plenty of fat and protein, there will be no shortage of fuel for the brain.

Whenever we're burning our own fat for fuel (which is, after all, what we want to do with it), our livers will also be taking some of this fat and converting it into ketones, and our brains will be using them for energy. This is a natural process. It happens any time we skip a meal and, most conspicuously, during the hours between dinner or late-night snack and breakfast, when our bodies live off the fat we stored during the day (or at least should be living off that fat). As the night goes on, we mobilize progressively more fat, and our livers up their production of ketones. By morning, we're technically in a state known as "ketosis," which means that our brains are primarily using ketones for fuel.* This is no

---

*Ketosis is often described by nutritionists as a "pathological" condition, but that's because they confuse ketosis with the ketoacidosis of uncontrolled diabetes. The former is natural; the latter is not. The ketone level in diabetic ketoacidosis typically exceeds 200 mg/dl, compared with the 5 mg/dl that we experience before our morning breakfast, and the 5 to 20 mg/dl of a severely carbohydrate-restricted diet.

different from what happens on a diet that restricts carbohydrates to fewer than sixty or so grams per day. Researchers have reported that the brain and central nervous system actually run more efficiently on ketones than they do on glucose.

In fact, we can define this mild ketosis as the normal state of human metabolism when we're not eating the carbohydrates that didn't exist in our diets for 99.9 percent of human history. As such, ketosis is arguably not just a natural condition but even a particularly healthful one. One piece of evidence in favor of this conclusion is that physicians have been using ketogenic diets to treat and even cure otherwise intractable childhood epilepsy since the 1930s. And researchers have recently taken to testing the idea that ketogenic diets can cure epilepsy in adults as well and even treat and cure cancer (an idea, as I'll discuss, that's not nearly as absurd as it might sound).

The Heart Disease Argument

This is the living-room elephant in any discussions of the risks or benefits of carbohydrate-restricted diets. Nutritionists initially got angry about carbohydrate restriction because they believed that the claims made for these diets were impossible, but this is the one that kept them angry and keeps their minds resolutely closed to any contrary evidence. They believe that if we buy into the logic of these diets, we'll replace what they consider "heart-healthy" carbohydrates—broccoli, whole-wheat bread, and potatoes, for instance—with meat, butter, eggs, and maybe cheese, which we very well might. Since the latter are all sources of saturated fat, the diets will raise our cholesterol, according to this logic, specifically the cholesterol in LDL (low-density lipoproteins), commonly known as the "bad" cholesterol, and we will have increased our risk of heart attack and premature death. This is the line of reasoning that prompted Jean Mayer to evoke his mass-murder metaphor. It's why most physicians and medical organizations still believe—or say they do—that the restricted carbohydrate diets are foolhardy.

There are many reasons to believe that they are wrong.

The first thing to question is the very idea that a diet that makes us lean by removing the fattening carbohydrates is also a diet that gives us heart disease. Recall Mayer's mass-murder argument: if we eat fewer carbohydrates, we'll replace those calories with fat. We will. Protein tends to stay in a narrow range in modern diets—15 to 25 percent of calories—whereas fat is traded off against carbohydrates: eating less of one means eating more of the other. If the one causes heart disease, then the other, almost by definition, has to prevent it. This is why carbohydrates became "heart-healthy" (even bread, pasta, potatoes, and sugar), and we were told to eat more of them when the authorities decided that eating fat clogged our arteries.

This would have little to do with the alleged evils of saturated fats except that there's a well-documented relationship between obesity and heart disease. Remember Blake Donaldson's "fat cardiacs"? Middle-aged men with a gut have always been obvious candidates for a heart attack. Fat, at least above the waist, and heart disease go hand in hand. (The fatter we are, or at least the more obese we are, the more likely we are to get virtually every major chronic disease.) That's why doctors are always urging their overweight patients to lose weight—even a little. The risk of having a heart attack should decrease significantly as a result.

So, if carbohydrates make us fat, which they do, and fat or saturated fat causes heart disease, which the authorities tell us they do, then we have a paradox: now the diet that naturally makes us leaner is also the diet that gives us heart disease. Getting leaner now increases our risk of heart disease, whereas it should do the opposite.

This paradox suggests that only one of these two things can be true: either carbohydrates make us fat *or* dietary fat gives us heart disease but not both. And, indeed, the fact that carbohydrates *do* make us fat—particularly, to repeat myself, easily digestible carbohydrates and sugars—suggests that these same carbohydrates are the likely nutritional causes of heart disease as well. This suggests that our obsession with the fat and saturated fat in our diets is simply misconceived.

Health authorities who insist that saturated fat causes heart disease have tried to escape this paradox—the diet that naturally makes us lean gives us heart disease—by blaming dietary fat for weight problems as well. They'll argue that fat is the most energy-dense nutrient in the diet, and this makes it fattening. It has nine calories per gram, compared with four for either protein or carbohydrates. Because of this high energy density, you are supposedly fooled more easily into overeating by fat than you are by the less dense calories of carbohydrates and protein. If you eat ten grams of fat for a midday snack, for instance, you'll be consuming fifty calories more than if you eat ten grams of protein or carbohydrates. Your body will care only about the ten grams, by this argument, not about the nutrients or the actual fuel available in those grams.

This idea is simplistic almost beyond belief. Imagine: hundreds of millions of years of evolution leading to organisms that determine how much fuel and essential nutrients they consume based only on the weight or energy density of the food, or the volume of the stomach cavity in which that food is digested. Not only is it hard to believe, but the experimental evidence has always refuted it. Even by the 1960s, high-fat, carbohydrate-restricted diets had been repeatedly shown to make people lose weight, not gain it. Still, by the 1970s, dietary fat had become the official dietary villain, and health authorities could now argue that saturated fat clogs our arteries and dietary fat in general makes us fat.

In 1984, this low-fat doctrine was officially set in stone when the National Heart, Lung, and Blood Institute (NHLBI) launched a "massive health campaign" to convince Americans that low-fat diets "will afford significant protection against coronary heart disease." The curious fact is that the NHLBI officials were actually less confident about the connection between dietary fat and heart disease than they were about the dietary fat/obesity idea. Here's how two of the leading experts in the science of cholesterol and heart disease—Nancy Ernst at the NHLBI, and Robert Levy, a former NHLBI director—described this logic at the time:

> There has been some indication that a low-fat diet decreases blood cholesterol levels. There is no conclusive proof that this lowering is independent of other concomitant changes in the diet. . . . It may be said with certainty, however, that because 1 g fat provides about 9 calories—compared to about 4 calories for 1 g of protein or carbohydrate—fat is a major source of calories in the American diet. Attempts to lose weight or maintain weight must obviously focus on the content of fat in the diet.

As a nation, we were told to eat less fat and less saturated fat, which we did, or at least tried to do—saturated-fat consumption steadily declined over the years that followed, according to U.S. Department of Agriculture statistics—and yet, rather than getting leaner, we got fatter.

What's more, the incidence of heart disease has not even diminished, which goes against expectations, if eating less fat or saturated fat makes a difference. This has been documented in numerous studies, the latest of which appeared in *The Journal of the American Medical Association* in November 2009 by Elena Kuklina and her colleagues at the Centers for Disease Control and Prevention. The authors made much of the fact that the number of Americans with high levels of LDL cholesterol has recently been decreasing, as would be expected in a nation avoiding saturated fat (and spending billions of dollars yearly on cholesterol-lowering drugs), but the number of heart attacks was not decreasing with it.

That the official embrace of low-fat, high-carbohydrate diets coincided not with a national decline in weight and heart disease but with epidemics of both obesity and diabetes (both of which increase heart disease risk), should make any reasonable person question the underlying assumptions of the advice. But that's not how people tend to think when confronted with evidence that one of their long-held beliefs is wrong. It's not how we typically deal with cognitive dissonance. It's certainly not how institutions and governments do it.

For the moment, I'll just say that the obesity/heart-disease link, combined with the obesity and diabetes epidemics that began more or less coincidentally with the advice to eat less fat, less saturated fat, and more carbohydrates, is a good reason to doubt that it's the fat and the saturated fat that we have to worry about.

Another reason to question the belief that saturated fat is bad for our health is that experimental evidence in support of the idea has always been surprisingly hard to come by. I know this seems difficult to believe, considering how forcefully we've been told that saturated fat is a killer. But what we've been told and what the evidence actually supports parted ways in 1984, when the National Heart, Lung, and Blood Institute launched its massive health campaign. At the time, the NHLBI experts lacked confidence in the fat/heart-disease connection, for good reason: the institute had spent $115 million on a huge, decade-long clinical trial to test the idea that eating less saturated fat would curb heart disease, but not a single heart attack had been prevented.*

This could have been taken as reason to abandon the idea entirely, but the institute had also spent $150 million testing the benefits of a cholesterol-lowering drug, and this second trial had succeeded. So the institute's administrators took a leap of faith, as

---

*The trial was known as the Multiple Risk Factor Intervention Trial. Eating less saturated fat was one of the multiple interventions tested. When the disappointing results were published in 1982, *The Wall Street Journal* headline said it all: "Heart Attacks, a Test Collapses."

one of them, Basil Rifkind, later described it: They had spent twenty years and an inordinate amount of money trying to demonstrate that cholesterol-lowering, low-fat diets would prevent heart disease, Rifkind explained, and they had, up until then, failed. Trying again would be too expensive and would take at least another decade, even if the institute could afford it. But once they had compelling evidence that lowering cholesterol with a drug would save lives, it seemed like a good bet that a low-fat, cholesterol-lowering diet would as well. "It's an imperfect world," Rifkind had said. "The data that would be definitive are ungettable, so you do your best with what is available."

The ambition was admirable, but the results have been, as I said, disappointing. Researchers have continued to demonstrate that cholesterol-lowering drugs can prevent heart attacks and apparently allow some people to live longer (at least those who are at particularly high risk of a heart attack). But it has still not been demonstrated that either low-fat or low-saturated-fat diets will do the same.

One problem here is that when people, experts or not, decide to review the evidence on an issue dear to their hearts (me included), they tend to see what they want to see. This is human nature, but it doesn't lead to trustworthy conclusions. To get around this problem, at least in medicine, an international organization was formed in the mid-1990s specifically to do *unbiased* reviews of the literature. This organization, known as the Cochrane Collaboration, is now widely considered to be among the most reliable sources for judgments about whether some intervention—a diet, a surgical procedure, a diagnostic technique— will actually do what doctors hope it does.

The Cochrane Collaboration assessed the benefits of eating less fat or less saturated fat in 2001. All told, the authors could find only twenty-seven clinical trials in the entire medical literature, dating back to the 1950s, that were conducted well enough so that a reliable judgment could be made about whether changing the fat content of our diet would prevent heart attacks and premature death. Many of the trials were actually designed to study whether these diets had effects on other conditions (such as breast cancer, hypertension, polyps, or gallstones), but the researchers who did the trials had also reported whether their subjects had heart attacks or died from them, and so the studies could be used to assess those issues as well. The evidence was anything but compelling.

"Despite decades of effort and many thousands of people randomized," the Cochrane Collaboration authors concluded, "there is still only limited and inconclusive evidence of the effects of modification of total, saturated, monounsaturated, or polyunsaturated fats on cardiovascular morbidity [i.e., sickness] and mortality [death]."

Since that Cochrane Collaboration analysis, the results of the largest, most expensive diet trial ever done have been published. That trial tested the benefits and risks of eating less fat and less saturated fat for women, who were rarely included in any of the earlier trials. This was the Women's Health Initiative that I mentioned back in chapter two. Forty-nine thousand middle-aged women were enrolled in the diet study, and twenty thousand of them were chosen at random to eat low-fat, low-saturated-fat diets, with less meat, more vegetables, more fresh fruits, and more whole grains. (This trial was funded not because the authorities were willing to doubt publicly that eating less fat would prevent heart disease but because previous trials had not included women, and the authorities were being pressured to take women's health as seriously as they did men's.)

After six years on the diet, these women had cut both their total fat consumption and their saturated-fat consumption by a quarter, lowering their total cholesterol and their LDL cholesterol below (albeit only very slightly below) that of the other twenty-nine thousand women, who were eating whatever they wanted and yet their low-fat diet, as the final reports stated, had *no* beneficial effect on heart disease, stroke, breast cancer, colon cancer, or, for that matter, fat accumulation. Eating less total fat and saturated fat, and replacing the fatty foods with fruits and vegetables and whole grains, had no observable beneficial effect at all.*

There are many problems with the kind of leap-of-faith, do-your-best, it's-a-good-bet logic that health authorities put into action in 1984, admirable and reasonable as it may have seemed at the time. The obvious one is that they will have our best interests in mind as they advise us to do something, but this something will end up doing more harm than good. The law of unintended consequences will take effect. In this case, we are told to eat less fat and more carbohydrates, and rather than avoid heart disease and get thinner, as the authorities had hoped we would, we've had as much heart disease as ever, and dramatic increases in obesity and diabetes.

A more insidious problem is that all involved—the researchers, the physicians, the public-health authorities, the health associations—commit themselves to a belief early in the evolution of the science, arguably at the stage at which they know the least about it, and then they become so invested in their belief that no amount of evidence to the contrary can convince them that they're wrong. As a result, when trials like the Women's Health Initiative find that eating less fat and less saturated fat has no beneficial effect (at least not for women), the authorities don't respond by acknowledging that they have made an error all along. Doing so might make them (and us) question their credibility, as it should. Instead, they tell us that the study must have been flawed, and thus the results can be ignored.

This is what happened with saturated fat. The belief that satu-

---

*In September 2009, the World Health Organization's Food and Agricultural Organization published a reassessment of the data on dietary fat and heart disease. "The available evidence from [observational studies] and randomized controlled trials," the report stated, "is unsatisfactory and unreliable to make judgment about and substantiate the effects of dietary fat on risk of CHD [coronary heart disease]."

rated fat clogs arteries by raising cholesterol levels is a hangover from the state of the science thirty to forty years ago. Back then, the evidence was poor, and it is still poor. But the belief was locked into the conventional wisdom, and still is, for a simple reason: LDL and total cholesterol are the two risk factors most obviously modified by cholesterol-lowering drugs, particularly statins (which are now worth billions of dollars yearly to the pharmaceutical industry). These drugs prevent heart attacks, and they may save lives. So the leap of faith is the same today as it was in 1984: if a drug that lowers cholesterol (and particularly LDL cholesterol) can prevent heart disease, then surely a diet that lowers cholesterol (and particularly LDL cholesterol) will prevent heart disease, whereas a diet that raises it must be a cause of heart disease. Saturated fat raises total cholesterol and LDL cholesterol. Ergo, saturated fat must cause heart disease, and diets that restrict saturated fat must prevent it.

This logic, though, has critical flaws. For starters, what drugs do and diets do are two entirely different things. Changing the nutrient content of our diets has many effects throughout our bodies, and many effects on different risk factors for heart disease, as do cholesterol-lowering drugs. That a particular fat in the diet raises LDL cholesterol, compared with, say, other fats or carbohydrates, does not mean it increases our risk of heart disease or is otherwise deleterious to our health.

Another flaw in the logic concerns the implication of causality: the fact that the drugs known as statins lower LDL cholesterol *and* prevent heart disease does not necessarily imply that they prevent heart disease *because* they lower LDL. Consider aspirin: it cures headaches *and* prevents heart disease, but no one would ever suggest that aspirin prevents heart disease *because* it cures headaches. It does other things as well, as statins do, and any one of these other things could be the reason why either drug prevents heart attacks.

.   .   .

When we consider all of the effects of the fats and carbohydrates in our diet, and all of the risk factors for heart disease that have become clear as the science has evolved since the 1970s, an entirely different picture emerges.

Let's start with triglycerides. These are also a risk factor for heart disease. The higher your level of circulating triglycerides (which are transported in the same lipoprotein particles that carry cholesterol), the greater the likelihood that you'll have a heart attack. This is not controversial. But it's the carbohydrates we eat that elevate triglyceride levels; fat, saturated or not, has nothing to do with them.

If you replace the saturated fat in your diet with carbohydrates—replace eggs and bacon for breakfast, say, with cornflakes, skim milk, and bananas—your LDL cholesterol may go down, but your triglycerides will go up. What *might* be a good thing, lowering LDL cholesterol (and I'll explain the "might" shortly), will be compensated for by a bad thing, raising triglycerides. This has been recognized since the early 1960s.

Low HDL cholesterol (aka the "good cholesterol") is also a risk factor for heart disease. Those of us with low HDL cholesterol are at far greater risk of having a heart attack than those of us with high total or LDL cholesterol. For women, HDL levels are so good at predicting future heart disease that they are, effectively, the only predictors of risk that matter. (When researchers look for genes that predispose individuals to living an exceedingly lengthy life—more than ninety-five or a hundred years—one of the few genes that stand out is a gene for a naturally high HDL cholesterol level.)

When you replace fat in your diet, even saturated fat, with carbohydrates, you lower your HDL, which means you make it more likely that you'll have a heart attack, at least by this predictor of risk. Once again, if you give up scrambled eggs and bacon for breakfast and replace them with cornflakes, skim milk, and bananas, your HDL cholesterol, your "good" cholesterol, will go *down*, and your heart-attack risk will go *up*. If you're currently eating cereal, skim milk, and bananas and switch instead to eggs and bacon, your HDL cholesterol will go up, and your heart-attack risk will go down. This has been known since the 1970s.

The advice we've been given to lower our total and LDL cholesterol *and* our body weight—eat less saturated fat and more carbohydrates—simply contradicts the advice we could have been given instead to raise our HDL, and HDL, again, is a far better predictor of heart disease. We've been told that we can increase our HDL by exercise, by losing weight, and even by moderate alcohol consumption, but we will rarely, if ever, be told that we can accomplish the same thing by replacing the carbohydrates in our diet with fat. (The reason why weight loss probably works so well to raise HDL is that the weight is lost—even on a low-calorie diet—because we eat fewer carbohydrates and less of the really fattening carbohydrates in particular. We lower our insulin levels, lose weight, *and* raise our HDL all because of the change in carbohydrate consumption.)

Nutritionists and public-health authorities who are resolute in their insistence that we eat low-fat, carbohydrate-rich diets to avoid heart disease will acknowledge in other contexts that carbohydrate-rich diets not only lower HDL cholesterol, and so increase our heart-disease risk, but do this so reliably that researchers have lately taken to using HDL as a way to determine the amount of carbohydrates that their clinical-trial subjects eat. HDL cholesterol, as a recent *New England Journal of Medicine* article explained, is "a biomarker for dietary carbohydrate."[*] In other words, if your HDL is high, it's a good bet that you're eating few carbohydrates. If your HDL cholesterol is low, then you're very likely eating a lot of carbohydrates.

---

[*]This was the trial of calorie-restricted diets carried out by researchers from Harvard and the Pennington Biomedical Research Center by Frank Sacks and his colleagues that I discussed in chapter 2. An editorial that accompanied the article in the *NEJM* explained the concept of HDL as a "biomarker for dietary carbohydrate" this way: "When fat is replaced isocalorically by carbohydrate, high-density lipoprotein (HDL) cholesterol decreases in a predictable fashion."

When we pay attention to how HDL tracks with heart disease—not just LDL and total cholesterol—we learn something about the purported risks and benefits of the foods we might choose to eat instead of fattening carbohydrates: red meat, say, or eggs and bacon, even lard and butter. It's important to understand that the fat in these foods is not all saturated. Rather, these animal fats are mixtures of saturated and unsaturated fats, just as vegetable fats are, and these fats all have different effects on our LDL and HDL cholesterol.

Take lard, for example, which has long been considered the archetypal example of a killer fat. It was lard that bakeries and fast-food restaurants used in large quantities before they were pressured to replace it with the artificial trans fats that nutritionists have now decided might be a cause of heart disease after all. You can find the fat composition of lard easily enough, as you can for most foods, by going to a U.S. Department of Agriculture website called the National Nutrient Database for Standard Reference. You'll find that nearly half the fat in lard (47 percent) is monounsaturated, which is almost universally considered a "good" fat. Monounsaturated fat raises HDL cholesterol *and* lowers LDL cholesterol (both good things, according to our doctors). Ninety percent of that monounsaturated fat is the same oleic acid that's in the olive oil so highly touted by champions of the Mediterranean diet. Slightly more than 40 percent of the fat in lard is indeed saturated, but a third of that is the same stearic acid that's in chocolate and is now also considered a "good fat," because it will raise our HDL levels but have no effect on LDL (a good thing and a neutral thing). The remaining fat (about 12 percent of the total) is polyunsaturated, which actually lowers LDL cholesterol but has no effect on HDL (also a good thing and a neutral thing).

In total, more than 70 percent of the fat in lard will improve your cholesterol profile compared with what would happen if you replaced that lard with carbohydrates. The remaining 30 percent will raise LDL cholesterol (bad) but also raise HDL (good). In other words, and hard as this may be to believe, if you replace the carbohydrates in your diet with an equal quantity of lard, it will actually reduce your risk of having a heart attack. It will make you healthier. The same is true for red meat, bacon and eggs, and virtually any other animal product we might choose to eat instead of the carbohydrates that make us fat. (Butter is a slight exception, because only half the fat will definitively improve your cholesterol profile; the other half will raise LDL but also raise HDL.)

Now let's look at what has happened in clinical trials in which subjects were instructed to do just what I've been proposing—replace the fattening carbohydrates they'd been eating with animal products high in fat and even high in saturated fat.

In the last ten years, researchers have carried out quite a few trials to compare diets that are very low in carbohydrates but high in fat and protein—typically, the Atkins diet, made famous by Dr. Robert Atkins in his 1972 best-seller, *Dr. Atkins' Diet Revolution*—with the kind of low-fat, low-calorie diet recommended by the American Heart Association or the British Heart Foundation.

These trials are the best studies ever done on the effect of eating high-fat, high-saturated-fat diets on weight and on risk factors for both heart disease and diabetes. The results have been remarkably consistent. In these trials, subjects would be instructed to eat as much fat and protein as they wanted—as much meat, fish, and fowl—but to avoid carbohydrates (eat fewer than fifty or sixty grams a day—200 to 240 calories' worth), and they would be compared with subjects who had been instructed not only to eat fewer total calories but particularly to avoid fat and saturated fat. This is what happened to those who ate mostly fat and protein:

1) They lost at least as much weight, if not considerably more.
2) Their HDL cholesterol went up.
3) Their triglycerides went way down.
4) Their blood pressure went down.
5) Their total cholesterol remained about the same.

6) Their LDL cholesterol went up slightly.
7) Their risk of having a heart attack decreased significantly.

Let's look at one of these studies in detail. This one cost two million dollars, was government-funded, and was done by researchers at Stanford University. The results were published in *The Journal of the American Medical Association* in 2007. It was known as the A TO Z Weight Loss Study and compared four diets:

1. The Atkins diet (A): twenty grams a day of carbohydrates for the first two to three months, and then fifty grams, with as much protein and fat as desired.
2. A traditional diet (T), also known as the LEARN diet (Lifestyle, Exercise, Attitudes, Relationships, and Nutrition): calories are restricted, carbohydrates make up 55 to 60 percent of all calories, fat is less than 30 percent, and saturated fat less than 10 percent. Regular exercise is encouraged.
3. The Ornish diet (O): fewer than 10 percent of all calories come from fat, and the subjects meditate and exercise.
4. The Zone diet (Z): 30 percent of calories come from protein, 40 percent from carbohydrates, and 30 percent from fat.

Here are the results for weight and for risk factors for heart disease, a year after the subjects embarked on their diets:

Group	Weight	LDL	Trig	HDL	BP*
Atkins	−9.9 lb	+ 0.8	−29.3	+4.9	−4.4
Traditional	−5.5 lb	+ 0.6	−14.6	−2.8	−2.2
Ornish	−5.3 lb	− 3.8	−14.9	0	−0.7
Zone	−3.3 lb	0	− 4.2	+2.2	−2.1

*Diastolic blood pressure.

Even though the subjects on the Atkins diet were counseled to eat as much food as they wanted, to eat copious amounts of red meat and thus the saturated fat that goes with it, they lost more weight, their triglycerides dropped further (a good thing), their HDL went up further (a good thing), and their blood pressure down further (a good thing) than those on any of the other diets.*

Here's how the Stanford researchers described the results:

> Many concerns have been expressed that low-carbohydrate weight-loss diets, high in total and saturated fat, will adversely affect blood lipid levels and cardiovascular risk. These concerns have not been substantiated in recent weight-loss diet trials. The recent trials, like the current study, have consistently reported that triglycerides, HDL-C [HDL cholesterol], blood pressure and measures of insulin resistance either were not significantly different or were more favorable for the very-low-carbohydrate groups.

The point man on this trial was Christopher Gardner, director of Nutrition Studies at the Stanford Prevention Research Center. Gardner presented the results of the trial in a lecture that's now viewable on YouTube — "The Battle of Weight Loss Diets: Is Anyone Winning (at Losing)?" He begins the lecture by acknowledging that he's been a vegetarian for twenty-five years. He did the study, he explains, because he was concerned that a diet like the Atkins diet, rich in meat and saturated fat, could be dangerous. When he described the triumph of the very low-carbohydrate, meat-rich Atkins diet, he called it "a bitter pill to swallow."

---

* The fact that the subjects only lost 10 pounds on the Atkins diet is not particularly telling as these people went back to eating significant carbohydrates as the study progressed. Their weight loss tracks with their carbohydrate consumption. At three months, they had lost 9 pounds and were reportedly eating an average of 240 to 250 calories of carbohydrates a day; at six months, 12 pounds and 450 calories of carbohydrates; at twelve months, only 10 pounds and 550 calories of carbohydrates.

The "Bad Cholesterol" Problem—
Updating the LDL Connection

These clinical trials alone should put your mind to rest about the idea that eating high-fat or high-saturated-fat diets will give you heart disease. But there are a few other factors worth discussing that most of these trials didn't address. The first involves LDL. It speaks again to how the science of heart disease has evolved since the 1970s.

When we first started hearing about the evils of LDL and physicians and health reporters began to refer to LDL as the "bad cholesterol," they did so because they thought it was the cholesterol that caused the buildup of plaque in our arteries. LDL, though, actually isn't cholesterol; it's the particle (the low-density lipoprotein—i.e., LDL) that contains the cholesterol and shuttles it (and triglycerides) around the bloodstream. The "bad cholesterol" terminology is a problem only because the researchers who study these things now say that it's not the cholesterol carried by the LDL that is to blame for heart disease but, rather, the LDL particle itself and other similar particles. The cholesterol seems to be an innocent bystander.

To complicate matters, not all LDL particles appear to be equally harmful, or "atherogenic," which is the term used by the experts to describe something that causes atherosclerosis or makes it worse. Some of the LDL in our circulation is large and buoyant, and some is small and dense, and there are gradations in between. The small and dense LDL particles appear to be the atherogenic ones, the ones we want to avoid. They work themselves into the walls of our arteries and begin the process of forming plaques. The large, buoyant LDL particles appear to be harmless.

This is important because carbohydrate-rich diets not only lower HDL and raise triglycerides, they also make LDL small and dense. These three effects all increase our risk of heart disease. When we eat high-fat diets and avoid carbohydrates, the opposite happens: HDL goes up, triglycerides go down, and the LDL in the circulation becomes larger and fluffier. Individually and together, these changes *decrease* our risk of having a heart attack. So what appears to be a bad thing, circa 1970 science (the effect of saturated fat on LDL cholesterol), is again a good thing, circa 2010 science (the effect of saturated fat on the LDL particle itself).

The health officials hesitate to discuss this science publicly, because it contradicts much of what we've been told for the past thirty to fifty years. Occasionally, though, researchers will let the facts break through, as did Chris Gardner and his Stanford colleagues when they wrote up the results of their A TO Z study. Their language is on the technical side, but it's not so technical that you shouldn't be able to follow it:

> Two of the more consistent findings in recent trials of low-carbohydrate vs low-fat diets have been higher [LDL cholesterol] concentrations and lower triglyceride concentrations in the low-carbohydrate diets. Although a higher [LDL cholesterol] concentration would appear to be an adverse effect, this may not be the case under these study conditions. The triglyceride-lowering effect of a low-carbohydrate diet leads to an increase in LDL particle size, which is known to decrease atherogenicity. In the current study, at 2 months, mean [LDL cholesterol] concentrations increased by 2% and mean triglyceride concentrations decreased by 30% in the Atkins group. These findings are consistent with a beneficial increase in LDL particle size, although LDL particle size was not assessed in our study.

These findings may indeed be a bitter pill for some to swallow, but they confirm that the diet we have to eat to lose weight—the one restricted in fattening carbohydrates—is also the diet that will best prevent heart disease.

Metabolic Syndrome

What I've tried to make clear in this chapter is that the fear of fat—saturated, in particular—is based on the state of the science in the 1960s and 1970s, and it simply doesn't hold up in the light of more recent research and the state of the science today. But one more very important point has to be made.

Earlier I discussed what happens when we become what's technically known as insulin-resistant—when muscle and liver cells, in particular, become resistant to the effect of the hormone insulin. Not only do we secrete more insulin in response, and so tend to get fatter, especially around the waist (where the fat cells are most sensitive to insulin), but we begin to manifest a host of other, related metabolic disturbances as well: blood pressure goes up; triglycerides go up; HDL cholesterol goes down. What I didn't mention earlier is that LDL particles become small and dense. We become glucose-intolerant, which means we have trouble controlling our blood sugar. We might even develop type 2 diabetes, which happens when the pancreas can no longer secrete enough insulin to compensate for the insulin resistance.

This combination of heart-disease risk factors is now known as "metabolic syndrome," and it is, in effect, the intermediate step on the way to heart disease. More than a quarter of the adult population in the United States now suffers from metabolic syndrome, according to the official estimates, and the reason why this number is so high is that metabolic syndrome includes diabetes and obesity among its symptoms, and we're experiencing epidemics of both. As you get fatter, as your waistline expands, you tend to lose control of your blood sugar; you are more likely to get hypertension, atherosclerosis, heart disease, and strokes. All these conditions are associated with the same cluster of what the experts call "lipid" abnormalities—low HDL, high triglycerides, and small, dense LDL. And all of these are triggered by the insulin resistance and the elevated insulin secretion that accompanies it, by the carbohydrates in our diet, and maybe the sugars (sucrose and high-fructose corn syrup) in particular.

The science of metabolic syndrome has been evolving since the late 1950s, when researchers first linked carbohydrate consumption to high triglycerides and then high triglycerides to heart disease. It went virtually unnoticed for decades because the heart-disease experts and the nutritionists were focused so obsessively on saturated fat and cholesterol. They didn't see a need to entertain alternative explanations for why we have heart attacks, and so they didn't. The driving force in the science of metabolic syndrome was a Stanford University physician named Gerald Reaven, who recognized early that excessive insulin secretion and insulin resistance are the root causes of this entire suite of metabolic disturbances.

When the authorities began paying attention to Reaven's work, in the mid-1980s, they had trouble embracing it, because his research implicated carbohydrates, not fat, as the dietary causes of both heart disease and diabetes. "Anyone who consumes more carbohydrates has to dispose of the load by secreting more insulin," as Reaven explained at a National Institutes of Health diabetes conference in 1986. Then he presented the evidence linking insulin to heart disease. The chair of the conference, Harvard's George Cahill, said Reaven's results "speak for themselves," which they did. But that was the problem. "Sometimes we wish it would go away, because nobody knows how to deal with it," said one NIH administrator of Reaven's work.

Today the science of metabolic syndrome represents probably the single greatest advance of the last half-century in our understanding of what causes heart disease and its intimate association with hypertension, obesity, and diabetes. It explains why those three conditions all increase dramatically our risk of heart disease, and why, if we have one of these conditions, we're likely to have the others as well. What metabolic syndrome tells us is that heart disease and diabetes are not caused by individual risk factors— low HDL, for instance, or high triglycerides, or small, dense

LDL—but by insulin resistance and elevated levels of insulin and blood sugar playing havoc with cells everywhere.

The insulin works on the fat cells to make us accumulate fat, and the expanding fat cells then release what are called "inflammatory molecules" ("cytokines," in the technical lingo) that have adverse effects throughout the body. It works on the liver to convert carbohydrates into fat, and this fat (triglycerides) is sent off into the bloodstream on the particles that eventually become small, dense LDL. It works on the kidney to raise blood pressure by reabsorbing sodium (and so has the same effect as eating extreme amounts of salt) and by impairing the secretion of uric acid, which also accumulates to unhealthy levels in the blood stream. (High uric-acid levels cause gout, which is also associated with obesity and diabetes, and the incidence of gout, too, is increasing in Western societies.) The insulin also works on the artery walls to stiffen them and cause the accumulation of triglycerides and cholesterol in the budding atherosclerotic plaques.

While this is happening, the chronically elevated blood sugar level that goes along with insulin resistance creates a host of problems on its own. It causes *oxidative stress* throughout the body. (The reason we're always told to consume foods rich with antioxidants is to combat or prevent this oxidative stress.) And it leads to the creation of *advanced glycation end products*, which seem to cause everything from the stiffening of our arteries to the aging of our skin and the premature aging that is part and parcel of diabetes.

To diagnose metabolic syndrome, doctors are told to look first for an expanding waistline, because metabolic syndrome is so closely tied to obesity. And because saying someone has metabolic syndrome is equivalent to saying someone is insulin-resistant, the experts blame both conditions on sedentary behavior and overeating. Why? Because they believe overeating and sedentary behavior make people fat. They then offer the familiar advice about low-fat diets (because they worry about the increased risk of heart disease that accompanies metabolic syndrome) and about eating less and exercising, because they think these are required for weight loss.

Here a little common sense is in order. As Reaven said a quarter-century ago, it's the carbohydrates that drive up insulin levels. We know now that carbohydrates make us fat, and it's been demonstrated in numerous clinical trials that low-carbohydrate, high-fat diets improve each and every one of the metabolic and hormonal abnormalities of metabolic syndrome—the low HDL, the high triglycerides, the small, dense LDL, the high blood pressure, and the insulin resistance and chronically elevated levels of insulin. This suggests the obvious: that the same carbohydrates that make us fat are the ones that cause metabolic syndrome. And it tells us that the best and perhaps only way to treat the condition, as with obesity and overweight, is to avoid carbohydrate-rich foods, particularly the ones we digest easily, and sugars.

Metabolic Syndrome Redux

Just a few more points need to be made about the importance of understanding the relationship between carbohydrates and metabolic syndrome. As it turns out, both Alzheimer's disease and most cancers—including breast cancer and colon cancer—are associated with metabolic syndrome, obesity, and diabetes. This means that, the fatter we are, the more likely we are to get cancer and the more likely we are to become demented as we age.* Researchers have begun to work out mechanisms through which insulin and high blood sugar might cause the brain deterioration

---

*David Schubert and Pamela Maher, neurobiologists at the Salk Institute for Biological Studies in San Diego, recently described the association with Alzheimer's this way: "There is a cluster of risk factors for Type 2 diabetes and vascular disease that include high blood glucose, obesity, high blood pressure, increased blood [triglycerides] and insulin resistance. All of these factors, both individually and collectively, increase the risk of Alzheimer's disease."

symptomatic of Alzheimer's (some researchers have even taken to referring to Alzheimer's as "type 3 diabetes") and how high blood sugar, insulin, and the related hormone, insulin-like growth factor, spur tumor growth and cause tumors to metastasize.

The link between cancer and metabolic syndrome is sufficiently well accepted that public-health recommendations have already been made based on this research. In 2007, the World Cancer Research Fund and the American Institute of Cancer Research jointly published a five-hundred-page report entitled *Food, Nutrition, Physical Activity and the Prevention of Cancer.* The report, co-authored by two dozen experts, discussed the evidence linking diet to cancer and found that the most convincing link ran from diet through "greater body fatness" to "cancers of the colorectum, esophagus (adenocarcinoma), pancreas, kidney and breast (postmenopause)," and probably gallbladder cancer as well.

The report then provided recommendations on how we might remain cancer free. The first is to "be as lean as possible" and "to avoid weight gain and increased waist circumference through adulthood." The second recommendation is to "be physically active as part of everyday life," because the experts who wrote this report believe that "physical activity protects against weight gain, overweight and obesity" and by doing so protects against cancer. And the third recommendation is to "limit consumption of energy-dense foods [and] avoid sugary drinks," because this is also thought "to prevent and control weight gain, overweight and obesity."

The first recommendation is now virtually indisputable. If you're lean, you will be less likely to get cancer than if you're obese. (Although this does *not* mean that body fatness causes cancers, as the report says.) The second and third recommendations are based on the belief that we get fat because we consume more calories than we expend. If the expert authors of the report had paid attention to the science of fat accumulation to Adiposity 101—nowhere to be found in the report's five hundred pages—

they would have concluded the obvious: that the same carbohydrates that make us fat are the ones that ultimately cause these cancers.

The simplest way to look at all these associations, between obesity, heart disease, type 2 diabetes, metabolic syndrome, cancer, and Alzheimer's (not to mention the other conditions that also associate with obesity and diabetes, such as gout, asthma, and fatty liver disease), is that what makes us fat—the quality and quantity of carbohydrates we consume—also makes us sick.

19

Following Through

This is not a diet book, because it's not a diet we're discussing. Once you accept the fact that carbohydrates—not overeating or a sedentary life—will make you fat, then the idea of "going on a diet" to lose weight, or what the health experts would call a "dietary treatment for obesity," no longer holds any real meaning. Now the only subjects worth discussing are how best to avoid the carbohydrates responsible—the refined grains, the starches, and the sugars—and what else we might do to maximize the benefits to our health.

Since the 1950s, some very thoughtful diet books have advocated that we restrict carbohydrates to control our weight, and these books have been appearing ever more frequently in recent years. Initially the authors were physicians, typically with weight problems themselves. This made their experiences similar: they failed to lose weight by eating less or exercising but eventually came upon the idea of restricting carbohydrates. They tried it, found that it worked, and prescribed it to their patients. Then they wrote books based on their experiences, both to get the message out and also to profit from whatever they considered their personal contribution to the genre. The books sold at first because the regimens worked and because there are always people who will try any new diet if they think it might work.

Eat Fat and Grow Slim (1958), *Calories Don't Count* (1960), *Dr. Atkins' Diet Revolution* (1972), *The Carbohydrate Addict's Diet* (1993), *Protein Power* (1996), and *Sugar Busters!* (1998) are all best-selling variations on the same theme: refined carbohydrates, starchy vegetables, and sugars are fattening; don't eat them, don't drink them.* These books are worth reading for the guidance they offer. But the diets themselves, no matter how they vary in the details or the author's understanding of the underlying science, fundamentally work because they restrict fattening carbohydrates.

In the appendix I have given a pared-down version of the kind of dietary guidelines that can be found in many books that would be classified as "low-carbohydrate" diets in bookstores or on websites. My directives are borrowed from the Lifestyle Medicine Clinic at the Duke University Medical Center (which in turn adapted them from the Atkins Center for Complementary Medicine). The clinic is run by Eric Westman, a physician who became intrigued by the diet in 1998, after one of his patients lost twenty pounds in two months and insisted he did so by eating large quantities of steak and little else. Westman responded by reading up on the Atkins diet, meeting with its author, Robert Atkins, in New York, and asking Atkins to fund a small pilot study (fifty patients, six months) to determine whether the diet works and is safe. The results confirmed that patients could lose weight and improve their cholesterol profiles on diets of virtually nothing but meat and leafy green vegetables.

Westman then visited physicians who were already using Atkins's diet in their clinics—Mary Vernon in Lawrence, Kansas; Richard Bernstein in Mamaroneck, New York; Joseph Hickey in Hilton Head, South Carolina; and Ron Rosedale in Boulder, Colorado—and reviewed their charts to verify that what Atkins was saying, and Westman's pilot study had concluded, actually

---

*The South Beach Diet (2003) is another best-selling variation on this theme, but with the emphasis on lean meats and fats from vegetable sources (olive and canola oil, avocados and nuts, for instance) rather than animal. In the one clinical trial of this diet, weight loss, as expected, rivaled the Atkins-like diets, but not the beneficial results for heart-disease and diabetes risk factors.

held up in clinical practice. In 2001, Westman began treating overweight and obese patients with the diet, and he's done so ever since. He has also continued to run clinical trials that have so far confirmed the health benefits of the diet—both in diabetics and in those without diabetes. (Westman is also an author, along with Stephen Phinney of the University of California, Davis, and Jeff Volek of the University of Connecticut, of the 2010 version of the Atkins diet book, *The New Atkins for a New You*.)

The guidelines that Westman distributes to his patients are more detailed but otherwise little different from the guidance offered by hospitals to their overweight and obese patients in the late 1940s and 1950s: Eat as much as you like of meat, fish, fowl, eggs, and leafy green vegetables. Avoid starches, grains, and sugars and anything made from them (including bread, sweets, juices, sodas), and learn for yourself whether and how much fruit and non-starchy vegetables (such as peas, artichokes, and cucumbers) your body can tolerate. If these concepts are familiar ones and the details are unnecessary, then I recommend taking the diet for obesity from Raymond Greene's 1951 endocrinology textbook, *The Practice of Endocrinology*, which I present on pages 155 and 156, and taping it to your refrigerator to refer to as necessary. If you need more details about which foods are acceptable and which are not, then the appendix is the better choice.

It would be nice if we could improve on the list of foods to eat, foods to avoid, and foods to eat in moderation. Unfortunately, this can't be done without guessing. The kind of long-term clinical trials have not been undertaken that would tell us more about what constitutes the healthiest variation of a diet in which the fattening carbohydrates have already been removed. We know from clinical trials that carbohydrate-restricted, eat-as-much-as-you-like diets work and that they have the expected beneficial effects on metabolic syndrome and thus our risk of heart disease. But that's the extent of the reliable knowledge so far.

What we have instead as a guide is the science itself—Adiposity 101—and the clinical experience of physicians like Westman who have had enough faith in their own observations and their understanding of the science to wean their overweight, obese, and diabetic patients off fattening carbohydrates, despite having to go against established convention to do so. From the experience of these physicians—Mary Vernon, Stephen Phinney, Jay Wortman of the University of British Columbia, and Michael and Mary Dan Eades, authors of *Protein Power*—I can offer a few thoughts on some of the obvious questions that are raised when we consider trading off fattening carbohydrates for a healthier and leaner life.

Moderation or Renounce Them Entirely? Part I

The fewer carbohydrates we consume, the leaner we will be. This is clear. But there's no guarantee that the leanest we *can* be will ever be as lean as we'd like. This is a reality to be faced. As I discussed, there are genetic variations in fatness and leanness that are independent of diet. Multiple hormones and enzymes affect our fat accumulation, and insulin happens to be the one hormone that we can consciously control through our dietary choices. Minimizing the carbohydrates we consume and eliminating the sugars will lower our insulin levels as low as is safe, but it won't necessarily undo the effects of other hormones—the restraining effect of estrogen that's lost as women pass through menopause, for instance, or of testosterone as men age—and it might not ultimately reverse all the damage done by a lifetime of eating carbohydrate- and sugar-rich foods.

This means that there's no one-size-fits-all prescription for the quantity of carbohydrates we can eat and still lose fat or remain lean. For some, staying lean or getting back to being lean might be a matter of merely avoiding sugars and eating the other carbohydrates in the diet, even the fattening ones, in moderation: pasta dinners once a week, say, instead of every other day. For others, moderation in carbohydrate consumption might not be sufficient, and far stricter adherence is necessary. And for some, weight will be lost only on a diet of virtually zero carbohydrates, and even this may not be sufficient to eliminate all our accumulated fat, or even most of it.

Whichever group you fall into, though, if you're not actively losing fat and yet want to be leaner still, the only viable option (short of surgery or the prospect that the pharmaceutical industry will come through with a safe and effective anti-obesity pill) is to eat still fewer carbohydrates, identify and avoid other foods that might stimulate significant insulin secretion—diet sodas, dairy products (cream, for instance), coffee, and nuts, among others— and have more patience. (Anecdotal evidence suggests that occasional or intermittent fasting for eighteen or twenty-four hours might work to break through these plateaus of weight loss, but this, too, has not been adequately tested.)

Physicians who have treated patients by prescribing carbohydrate-restricted diets for a decade or longer and published discussions of their clinical experiences—the British physician Robert Kemp, for instance, who began doing so in 1956, and Wolfgang Lutz, an Austrian physician, who began a year later— have reported that a small proportion of their obese patients failed to lose any significant fat even though they faithfully avoid fattening carbohydrates (or at least said they did). Women failed more often than men, and older patients more often than younger ones. The more obese the patients, and the longer they had been obese, the more likely they were to remain obese.* However, as Lutz said, this doesn't mean "that the carbohydrates were not responsible for the disorder [obesity] in the first place. It is quite simply, and sadly, that a point of no return has been reached."

---

*Kemp discussed his experience in a series of three articles published in the British medical journal *Practitioner* between 1963 and 1972, by which time he'd treated almost fifteen hundred obese and overweight patients. Lutz discussed his results in his 1967 book *Leben ohne Brot (Life Without Bread)*, which was republished in English and revised with the help of Christian Allan, a biochemist, in 2000.

What we don't know is whether these individuals could have succeeded had they further restricted carbohydrates, or had they simply had more patience, and maybe both. The conventional logic of diets is that people go on them expecting relatively quick returns in weight loss. By this logic, the dieters are not trying to reregulate their fat tissue; they're only reducing the calories they consume, with the expectation that their fat cells will willingly respond by giving up the calories they've sequestered. If dieters see no significant losses in a month or two, they decide that the diet has failed and either move to the next one or resign themselves to their adiposity. But the fact is that we *are* trying to counteract a regulatory disorder of fat metabolism, one that may have been years or decades in the making. Reversing the process might take more than a few months or even a few years as well.

Carbohydrate restriction is often equated with eating animals and animal products. The reason is simple: if you eat mostly plants or exclusively plants, you're getting the bulk of your calories from carbohydrates, by definition. This doesn't mean that you can't become lean or remain lean by giving up sugars, flour, and starchy vegetables, and living exclusively on leafy green vegetables, whole grains, and pulses (beans). But it is unlikely to work for many of us, if not most. Leafy green vegetables and pulses have the advantage that the carbohydrates they contain aren't digested quickly—they have what nutritionists call a low glycemic index—but if you're relying on these foods for the bulk of your diet, then the total amount of carbohydrates you're consuming (the glycemic load of your diet) will still be high. This may be enough either to make you fat or to keep you fat. If you try to eat fewer carbohydrates by eating smaller portions, you'll be hungry, with all the problems that entails.

So if you are a vegan or a vegetarian you can still benefit from an understanding of Adiposity 101. You can always improve the quality of the carbohydrates you eat, even if you don't reduce the total quantity. This change alone will assuredly improve your health, even if it's not sufficient to make you lean.

Moderation or Renounce Them Entirely? Part II

Over the years, the physicians promoting carbohydrate restriction have typically taken one of three approaches to maximizing the effect and the sustainability (equally important) of this manner of eating.

One is to establish an ideal amount of carbohydrates that you can and perhaps should eat—say, the seventy-two grams a day, or nearly three hundred calories' worth, that Wolfgang Lutz prescribes. This is intended to minimize any potential side effects that might occur when the body makes the transition from burning primarily carbohydrates for fuel to burning fat. The approach also assumes that it's easier to eat some fattening carbohydrates than it is to eliminate them entirely. With this logic, Lutz allows "small amounts of sugar and an occasional dessert, some crumbs for breaded food, a little lactose (in milk), and small quantities of carbohydrate in vegetables and fruit." This may work for some of us but not for all.

Another approach is to aim for minimal carbohydrates from the outset. You don't need them in your diet, so this logic goes, and any short-term side effects you might experience while your body adjusts to a nearly carbohydrate-free diet can be managed (more on that).

The third option is a compromise that was pioneered by Robert Atkins forty years ago. It was based on what seems like an obvious point to make (although not so obvious that the health experts today tend to make it): You enter into a weight-loss diet with the singular purpose of becoming as lean as you safely can be, and so all other gustatory desires should be put on hold *temporarily* until that goal is achieved. When you have achieved your goal and the excess fat has been lost, you can decide if you feel the need to incorporate back into your diet some of the foods you've been avoiding.

Diets that operate on this philosophy typically begin with what Atkins called an "induction phase," which allows effectively no carbohydrates (fewer than twenty grams a day in Atkins's diet). This has the effect of accelerating initial weight loss and providing encouragement to stick with the diet. You're instructed to give up all carbohydrates, with the sole exception of a few small portions of leafy green vegetables each day. Once your body is actively engaged in burning its own fat stores and you're losing weight at an acceptable pace, a minimal amount of carbohydrates can be added back into the diet. If, however, you stop losing fat, that means your body can't tolerate these carbohydrates and you can't eat them.

The same approach can be used once an ideal weight is reached. Add back whatever carbohydrate-rich foods you particularly miss and see how your body responds. If you begin to gain weight, say, because you're now eating an apple a day, and you don't want to be any heavier, then don't eat the apple. If you don't gain weight, that means your body can tolerate an apple a day, and you can experiment with other carbohydrates. You can see what happens when you also eat an orange a day or a pasta dinner once a week or the occasional dessert. This allows you to determine what your body can tolerate and how much fat you're willing to accommodate for the foods you miss.

This approach makes sense. But one other factor has to be taken into account: allowing some carbohydrates into the diet for some individuals may be like allowing ex-smokers a few cigarettes or reformed alcoholics the occasional drink.* Some may be able to deal with it; some may find it is a slippery slope. The occasional

---

*In *The Carbohydrate Addict's Diet* Rachel and Richard Heller argue, in effect, the exact opposite: that sustained weight loss is best achieved by eating one balanced "Reward Meal" a day that includes carbohydrates. This is another concept that may be true and is worth a try, but has never been adequately tested.

dessert on special occasions may become a weekly luxury, then biweekly, and finally nightly, and suddenly you've decided that carbohydrate restriction failed as a weight-loss regimen because you failed to stick with it and regained the weight.

A common argument that many experts wield against carbo-hydrate restriction is that *all* diets fail, the reason being that people just don't stay on diets. So why bother? But this argument implicitly assumes that all diets work in the same way—we consume fewer calories than we expend—and thus all fail in the same way.

But this isn't true. If a diet requires that you semi-starve yourself, it will fail, because (1) your body adjusts to the caloric deficit by expending less energy, (2) you get hungry and stay hungry, and (3), a product of both of these, you get depressed, irritable, and chronically tired. Eventually you go back to eating what you always did—or become a binge eater—because you can't abide semi-starvation and *its* side effects indefinitely.

When you restrict fattening carbohydrates, however, you don't have to restrict consciously how much you eat; indeed, you shouldn't try. You can eat all you want of protein and fat, so you don't get hungry and you don't expend less energy. You might even expend more. The biggest challenge is the craving for car-bohydrates. The hunger that accompanies our attempts to eat fewer calories is an unavoidable physiological phenomenon; the craving for carbohydrates is more like an addiction. It is the consequence, at least in part, of insulin resistance and the chronically elevated levels of insulin that go with it, and thus caused by the carbohydrates in the first place.

Sugars are a special case. As I discussed earlier, sugar appears to be addictive in the brain in the same way in which cocaine, nicotine, and heroin are. This suggests that the relatively intense cravings for sugar—a sweet tooth—may be explained by the intensity of the dopamine secretion in the brain when we consume sugar.

Whether the addiction is in the brain or the body or both, the idea that sugar and other easily digestible carbohydrates are addictive also implies that the addiction can be overcome if you make the effort and have sufficient patience. This is not the case with hunger itself. Avoiding carbohydrates will lower your insulin level. Given time, this should reduce or eliminate the cravings. It could, however, take longer than you'd expect or ideally like. In 1975, the Duke University pediatrician James Sidbury, Jr. (who would become director that same year of the National Institute of Child Health and Human Development at the National Institutes of Health), reported great success slimming down obese children on a diet of only 15 percent carbohydrates. "After a year to 18 months," he wrote, "the craving for sweets is lost," and the children often pinpointed when this happened to "within a specific one to two week period."

If you continue to eat some of the fattening carbohydrates or allow yourself some sugar (or even, perhaps, artificial sweeteners), though, you may always have the cravings. You may always have what Stephen Phinney refers to as "intrusive thoughts of food." Anecdotal evidence suggests this is the case, and that's all we have to go on.

The implication is that for some, at least, long-term success may be more likely if no compromise is allowed. If you do compromise and eventually return to eating these carbohydrates in quantity, the only reasonable response if weight loss remains your goal will be to try again, just as smokers might try to quit numerous times before they ultimately succeed. There's no other viable option when you find yourself eating fattening carbohydrates again and regaining weight. Try to quit again, or at least cut back to some minimal level.

What It Means to Eat as Much as We Would Like

If you have grown up with one belief system (with one paradigm, as sociologists of science say), it's hard to leave it behind entirely when you open your mind to accept another. We've been told for so long, and believed for so long, that a fundamental requirement for weight loss is that we eat less than we'd like, and for weight maintenance that we eat in moderation, that it's natural to assume the same is true when we restrict the carbohydrates we eat. Eating less of everything, though, as I discussed earlier, is another way of saying that we're going to restrict consciously the amount of protein and fat we consume, as well as the carbohydrates. But protein and fat don't make us fat—only the carbohydrates do—so there is no reason to curtail them in any way.

It's true that people who restrict carbohydrates often eat less than they otherwise might. A common experience is to give up fattening carbohydrates and find that you're not as hungry as you used to be, that mid-morning snacks are no longer necessary. Intrusive thoughts of food and the urge to satisfy them vanish. But that's because you're now burning your fat stores for fuel, which you didn't do before. Your fat cells are now working properly as short-term energy buffers, not long-term lockups for the calories they've sequestered. You have an internal supply of fuel that keeps you going throughout the day and night, as it should, and your appetite adjusts accordingly. If you're not running short on fuel, you feel no need to restock every few hours. (If you're losing two pounds a week, that's seven thousand calories of your own fat that you're burning for fuel every week—one thousand calories each day that you don't have to eat.)

Another effect, though, of restricting carbohydrates is that your energy expenditure should increase. You're no longer diverting fuel into your fat tissue, where you can't use it, and so you literally have more energy to burn. By avoiding the fattening carbohydrates, you remove the force that diverts calories into your fat cells. Your body should then find its own balance between energy consumed (appetite and hunger) and energy expended (physical activity and metabolic rate). This process could take time, but it should happen without conscious thought.

Trying to rein in appetite consciously could lead to compensatory responses. You might have less energy to burn, so your energy expenditure won't increase, or you hold on to fat that you'd otherwise burn. You might lose lean tissue (muscle) that you might otherwise maintain. And the conscious self-restraint might prompt an urge to binge. Physicians who prescribe carbohydrate restrictions in their clinics say that their patients get the best results when they're reminded or urged to eat whenever they're hungry and until they're satisfied or even to schedule snacks every few hours and eat whether they are hungry or not.

The same argument holds for exercise. There are very good reasons to be physically active, but weight loss, as I discussed earlier, does not appear to be one of them. Exercise will make you hungry, and it's likely to reduce your energy expenditure during times when you're not exercising. The goal is to avoid both of these responses. Trying to drive weight loss by increasing energy expenditure may be not only futile but also actively counterproductive. You tend to be sedentary when you're overweight or obese because of the partitioning of fuel into your fat tissue that you could be burning for energy. You literally lack the energy to exercise, and so the impulse to do it. Once that problem is fixed— by avoiding the carbohydrates that made you and keep you fat— then you should have the energy to be physically active and with it the drive or impulse to do so.

The goal is to remove the cause of your excess adiposity—the fattening carbohydrates—and let your body find its own natural equilibrium between energy expenditure and consumption. So you should eat when you're hungry and eat until you're full. If you're not eating carbohydrate-rich foods, you won't get fat or fatter by doing so. Once you start burning your own fat for fuel, you should have the energy to be physically active as well.

Fat or Protein?

Another hangover from the last half-century of dietary misguidance is the belief that dietary fat must indeed be bad for us, even if we accept that carbohydrates are causing us to fatten.

This is a compromise position that seems perfectly reasonable. It was this kind of thinking in the early 1960s that led proponents of carbohydrate restriction to describe their recommended diets as high in protein instead of high in fat. Rather than avoiding only the fattening carbohydrates, you eliminate butter and cheese from the diet, eat chicken breasts without the skin, lean fish, the leanest cuts of meat, and egg whites without the yolks.

As I've said, though, there's no compelling reason to think that fat, or saturated fat, is harmful, whereas there's good reason to question the benefits of diets that abnormally elevate the protein content. Populations that ate mostly meat or exclusively meat, as I discussed earlier, tried to maximize the fat they ate, and one reason seems to be that high-protein diets—without significant fat or carbohydrates—can be toxic. This issue has been addressed by protein-metabolism experts in a recent U.S. Institute of Medicine Report called *Dietary Reference Intakes*.

"It has been suggested from evidence of the dietary practices of hunter-gatherer populations, both present day and historical, that humans avoid diets that contain too much protein," the IOM experts explain, citing the same research on hunter-gatherer populations to which I referred. The short-term symptoms of these high-protein, *low-fat*, low-carbohydrate diets, these protein-metabolism experts point out, are weakness, nausea, and diarrhea. These symptoms will disappear when the protein content is reduced to a more moderate 20 to 25 percent of calories and fat content is increased to compensate.

When physicians and nutritionists tested carbohydrate restriction before the beginning of the anti-fat movement in the 1960s, they did so with fatty meat and diets that were 75 to 80 percent fat by calories but only 20 to 25 percent protein. This mixture had no side effects, was well tolerated, and is most consistent with the diets eaten by populations like the Inuits, who lived almost exclusively, if not exclusively, on animal products.

Whether or not a diet that is 75 percent fat and 25 percent protein is healthier than one that is 65 percent fat and 35 percent protein is an open question. Equally important is the question of which is easier to sustain and provides the most enjoyment. If you find yourself satisfied eating skinless chicken breasts, lean cuts of meat and fish, and egg-white omelets, so be it. But eating the fat of the meat as well as the lean, the yolk as well as the white, foods cooked with butter and lard may be the better prescription for sustainability, and it may be for health as well.

On Side Effects and Doctors

When you replace the carbohydrates you eat with fat, you're creating a radical shift in the fuel that your cells will burn for energy. They go from running primarily on carbohydrates (glucose) to running on fat—both your body fat and the fat in your diet. This shift, though, can come with side effects. These can include weakness, fatigue, nausea, dehydration, diarrhea, constipation, a condition known as postural, or orthostatic, hypotension—if you stand up too quickly, your blood pressure drops precipitously, and you can get dizzy or even pass out—and the exacerbation of pre-existing gout. In the 1970s, the authorities insisted that these "potential side effects" were reasons why the diets could not "generally be used safely," and the implication was that they shouldn't be used at all.

But that was to confuse the short-term effects of what can be thought of as carbohydrate withdrawal with the long-term benefits of overcoming that withdrawal and living a longer, leaner, and healthier life. The more technical term for carbohydrate withdrawal is "keto-adaptation," because the body is adapting to the state of ketosis that results from eating fewer than sixty or so grams of carbohydrates a day. This reaction is why some who try carbo-hydrate restriction give it up quickly.* ("Carbohydrate withdrawal is often interepreted as a 'need for carbohydrate,' " says Westman. "It's like telling smokers who are trying to quit that their with-drawal symptoms are caused by a 'need for cigarettes' and then suggesting they go back to smoking to solve the problem.")

The reason for the side effects now appears to be clear, and physicians who prescribe carbohydrate restriction say they can be treated and prevented. These symptoms have nothing to do with the high fat content of the diet. Rather, they appear to be a conse-quence of either eating too much protein and too little fat, of attempting strenuous exercise without taking the time to adapt to the diet, or, in most cases, of the body's failure to compensate fully for the restriction of carbohydrates and the dramatic lower-ing of insulin levels that ensues.

As I mentioned in passing earlier, insulin signals our kidneys to reabsorb sodium, which in turn causes water retention and raises blood pressure. When insulin levels drop, as they do when we restrict carbohydrates, our kidneys will excrete the sodium they've been retaining and with it water. For most people this is beneficial, and it's the reason why blood pressure comes down with carbohydrate restriction. (This water loss, which can be a half-dozen pounds or more in a two-hundred-pounder, can con-stitute most of the early weight loss.) For some individuals, though, the body will perceive the water loss as something to be prevented. It does so through a web of compensatory responses that can lead to water retention and what are called electrolyte

---

*The same is true for the occasional elevation of cholesterol that will occur with fat loss—"transient hypercholesterolemia"—a consequence of the fact that we store cholesterol along with fat in our fat cells. When fatty acids are mobi-lized, the cholesterol is released as well, and cholesterol levels can spike as a result. The existing evidence suggests that cholesterol levels will return to nor-mal, or fall even lower than what they were, once the excess fat is lost—regardless of the saturated-fat content of the diet.

imbalances (the kidneys excrete potassium to save sodium), and the result is the side effects just cited. The reaction can be countered, as Phinney has noted, by adding sodium back into the diet: taking a gram or two of sodium a day (a half to one teaspoon of salt) or drinking a couple of cups of chicken or beef broth daily, which is what Westman, Vernon, and other physicians now prescribe.

These side effects speak to the importance of having the guidance of a knowledgeable physician when making the decision to avoid fattening carbohydrates. If you happen to be diabetic or hypertensive, then a doctor's guidance is critical. Since restricting carbohydrates will lower both blood sugar and blood pressure, if you're already taking drugs to do the same, the combination can be dangerous. Abnormally low blood sugar (known as hypoglycemia) can cause seizures, unconsciousness, and even death. Abnormally low blood pressure (hypotension) can induce dizziness, fainting, and seizures.

Doctors who understand why we get fat and what to do about it are obviously hard to find; otherwise, this book wouldn't be necessary. The truly unfortunate fact is that even those doctors who do understand the reality of weight regulation often hesitate to prescribe carbohydrate restriction to their patients—even if this is how they maintain their own weight. Physicians who tell their fat patients to eat less and exercise more, and particularly to eat the kind of low-fat, high-carbohydrate diet that the authorities recommend, will not be sued for malpractice should any of those patients have a heart attack two weeks or even two months later. The doctor who goes against established medical convention and prescribes carbohydrate restriction has no such safeguard.*

---

*As Blake Donaldson said in his 1962 memoirs, no matter how well someone does on the mostly meat diet that Donaldson prescribed, "any disaster that may overtake him, even to the extent of ground moles getting in his lawn, will be blamed on his diet."

There are now innumerable diet books that preach carbohydrate restriction, not to mention cookbooks and websites devoted to low-carbohydrate eating, and even smart-phone apps that can be used for guidance. But it's vital that doctors understand what I've discussed here, that they open their minds to these ideas and, more important, to the hard science that has too often been ignored. This is true of public-health officials, too, not to mention the obesity researchers themselves. As long as these authorities buy into the logic of calories-in/calories-out and dismiss carbohydrate restriction as a fad diet, we will suffer for it. We need their help, which is why this book was written as much for your doctors as for you. Until our doctors truly understand why we get fat, and until our public-health authorities do, the job of losing that fat and remaining healthy will always be far more difficult than it need be.

APPENDIX

Lifestyle Medicine Clinic
Duke University Medical Center

"No Sugar, No Starch" Diet: Getting Started

This diet is focused on providing your body with the nutrition it needs, while eliminating foods that your body does not require, namely, nutritionally empty carbohydrates. For most effective weight loss, you will need to keep the total number of carbohydrate grams to *fewer than 20 grams per day*. Your diet is to be made up exclusively of foods and beverages from this handout. If the food is packaged, check the label and make sure that the carbohydrate count is 1 to 2 grams or less for meat and dairy products, 5 grams or less for vegetables. All food may be cooked in a microwave oven, baked, boiled, stir-fried, sautéed, roasted, fried (with no flour, breading, or cornmeal), or grilled.

WHEN YOU ARE HUNGRY,
EAT YOUR CHOICE OF THE FOLLOWING FOODS:

Meat: Beef (including hamburger and steak), pork, ham (unglazed), bacon, lamb, veal, or other meats. For processed meats (sausage, pepperoni, hot dogs), check the label—carbohydrate count should be about 1 gram per serving.

Poultry: Chicken, turkey, duck, or other fowl.

Fish and Shellfish: Any fish, including tuna, salmon, catfish, bass, trout, shrimp, scallops, crab, and lobster.

Eggs: Whole eggs are permitted without restrictions.

Appendix

You do not have to avoid the fat that comes with the above foods.

You do not have to limit quantities deliberately, but you should stop eating when you feel full.

FOODS THAT MUST BE EATEN EVERY DAY:

Salad Greens: *2 cups a day.* Includes arugula, bok choy, cabbage (all varieties), chard, chives, endive, greens (all varieties, including beet, collards, mustard, and turnip), kale, lettuce (all varieties), parsley, spinach, radicchio, radishes, scallions, and watercress. (If it is a leaf, you may eat it.)

Vegetables: *1 cup (measured uncooked) a day.* Includes artichokes, asparagus, broccoli, Brussels sprouts, cauliflower, celery, cucumber, eggplant, green beans (string beans), jicama, leeks, mushrooms, okra, onions, peppers, pumpkin, shallots, snow peas, sprouts (bean and alfalfa), sugar snap peas, summer squash, tomatoes, rhubarb, wax beans, zucchini.

Bouillon: *2 cups daily—as needed for sodium replenishment.* Clear broth (consommé) is strongly recommended, unless you are on a sodium-restricted diet for hypertension or heart failure.

FOODS ALLOWED IN LIMITED QUANTITIES:

Cheese: *up to 4 ounces a day.* Includes hard, aged cheeses such as Swiss and Cheddar, as well as Brie, Camembert, blue, mozzarella, Gruyère, cream cheese, goat cheeses. Avoid processed cheeses, such as Velveeta. Check the label; carbohydrate count should be less than 1 gram per serving.

Cream: *up to 4 tablespoonfuls a day.* Includes heavy, light, or sour cream (not half and half).

Mayonnaise: *up to 4 tablespoons a day.* Duke's and Hellmann's are low-carb. Check the labels of other brands.

Olives (Black or Green): *up to 6 a day.*

Avocado: *up to 1/2 of a fruit a day.*

Lemon/Lime Juice: *up to 4 teaspoonfuls a day.*

Soy Sauces: *up to 4 tablespoons a day.* Kikkoman is a low-carb brand. Check the labels of other brands.

Pickles, Dill or Sugar-Free: *up to 2 servings a day.* Mt. Olive makes sugar-free pickles. Check the labels for carbohydrates and serving size.

Snacks: Pork rinds/skins; pepperoni slices; ham, beef, turkey, and other meat roll-ups; deviled eggs.

THE PRIMARY RESTRICTION: CARBOHYDRATES

On this diet, no sugars (simple carbohydrates) and no starches (complex carbohydrates) are eaten. The only carbohydrates encouraged are the nutritionally dense, fiber-rich vegetables listed.

Sugars are simple carbohydrates. *Avoid these kinds of foods:* white sugar, brown sugar, honey, maple syrup, molasses, corn syrup, beer (contains barley malt), milk (contains lactose), flavored yogurts, fruit juice, and fruit.

Starches are complex carbohydrates. *Avoid these kinds of foods:* grains (even "whole" grains), rice, cereals, flour, cornstarch, breads, pastas, muffins, bagels, crackers, and "starchy" vegetables such as slow-cooked beans (pinto, lima, black beans), carrots, parsnips, corn, peas, potatoes, French fries, potato chips.

FATS AND OILS

All fats and oils, even butter, are allowed. Olive oil and peanut oil are especially healthy oils and are encouraged in cooking. Avoid margarine and other hydrogenated oils that contain trans fats.

For salad dressings, the ideal dressing is a homemade oil-and-vinegar dressing, with lemon juice and spices as needed. Blue-cheese, ranch, Caesar, and Italian are also acceptable if the label says 1 to 2 grams of carbohydrate per serving or less. Avoid "lite" dressings, because these commonly have more carbohydrates. Chopped eggs, bacon, and/or grated cheese may also be included in salads.

Fats, in general, are important to include, because they taste good and make you feel full. You are therefore permitted the fat or skin that is served with the meat or poultry that you eat, as long as there is no breading on the skin. *Do not attempt to follow a low-fat diet!*

SWEETENERS AND DESSERTS

If you feel the need to eat or drink something sweet, you should select the most sensible alternative sweetener(s) available. Some available alternative sweeteners are: Splenda (sucralose), Nutra-sweet (aspartame), Truvia (stevia/erythritol blend), and Sweet 'N Low (saccharin). Avoid food with sugar alcohols (such as sorbitol and maltitol) for now, because they occasionally cause stomach upset, although they may be permitted in limited quantities in the future.

BEVERAGES

Drink as much as you would like of the allowed beverages, but do not force fluids beyond your capacity. The best beverage is water. Essence-flavored seltzers (zero carbs) and bottled spring and mineral waters are also good choices.

Caffeinated beverages: Some patients find that their caffeine intake interferes with their weight loss and blood sugar control. With this in mind, you may have *up to 3 cups of coffee* (black, or with artificial sweetener and/or cream), tea (unsweetened or artificially sweetened), or caffeinated diet soda per day.

Appendix

ALCOHOL

At first, avoid alcohol consumption on this diet. At a later point in time, as weight loss and dietary patterns become well established, alcohol in moderate quantities, if low in carbohydrates, may be added back into the diet.

QUANTITIES

Eat when you are hungry; stop when you are full. The diet works best on a "demand feeding" basis—that is, eat whenever you are hungry; try not to eat more than what will satisfy you. Learn to listen to your body. A low-carbohydrate diet has a natural appetite-reduction effect to ease you into the consumption of smaller and smaller quantities comfortably. Therefore, do not eat everything on your plate just because it's there. On the other hand, don't go hungry! You are not counting calories. Enjoy losing weight comfortably, without hunger or cravings.

It is recommended that you start your day with a nutritious low-carbohydrate meal. Note that many medications and nutritional supplements need to be taken with food at each meal, or three times per day.

IMPORTANT TIPS AND REMINDERS

The following items are NOT on the diet: sugar, bread, cereal, flour-containing items, fruits, juices, honey, whole or skimmed milk, yogurt, canned soups, dairy substitutes, ketchup, sweet condiments and relishes.

Avoid these common mistakes: Beware of "fat-free" or "lite" diet products, and foods containing "hidden" sugars and starches (such as coleslaw or sugar-free cookies and cakes). Check the labels of liquid medications, cough syrups, cough drops, and other over-the-counter medications that may contain sugar. Avoid products that are labeled "Great for Low-Carb Diets!"

LOW-CARB MENU PLANNING

What does a low-carbohydrate menu look like? You can plan your daily menu by using the following as a guide:

Breakfast
Meat or other protein source (usually eggs)

Fat source—*This may already be in your protein; for example, bacon and eggs have fat in them. But if your protein source is "lean," add some fat in the form of butter, cream (in coffee), or cheese.*

Low-carbohydrate vegetable (if desired)—*This can be in an omelet or a breakfast quiche.*

Lunch
Meat or other protein source

Fat source—*If your protein is "lean," add some fat, in the form of butter, salad dressing, cheese, cream, or avocado.*

1 to 1½ cups of salad greens or cooked greens

½ to 1 cup of vegetables

Snack
Low-carbohydrate snack that has protein and/or fat

Dinner
Meat or other protein source

Fat source—*If your protein is "lean," add some fat in the form of butter, salad dressing, cheese, cream, or avocado.*

1 to 1½ cups of salad greens or cooked greens

½ to 1 cup of vegetables

A sample day may look like this:

Breakfast
Bacon or sausage

Eggs

Lunch
Grilled chicken on top of salad greens and other vegetables, with
bacon, chopped eggs, and salad dressing

Snack
Pepperoni slices and a cheese stick

Dinner
Burger patty or steak
Green salad with other acceptable vegetables and salad dressing
Green beans with butter

READING A LOW-CARB LABEL

Start by checking the nutrition facts.

- Look at serving size, total carbohydrate, and fiber.
- Use total carbohydrate content only.
- You may subtract fiber from total carbohydrate to get the
  "effective or net carb count." For example, *if there are 7
  grams of carbohydrate and 3 grams of fiber, the difference
  yields 4 grams of effective carbohydrates.* That means the
  effective carbohydrate count is 4 grams per serving.
- No need to worry—at this point—about calories or fat.
- Effective carbohydrate count of vegetables should be 5
  grams or less.
- Effective carbohydrate count of meat or condiments should
  be 1 gram or less.
- Also check the ingredient list. Avoid foods that have any
  form of sugar or starch listed in the first 5 ingredients.

Sugar by any other name is still sugar!
All of these are forms of sugar: sucrose, dextrose, fructose, maltose, lactose, glucose, honey, agave syrup, high-fructose corn
syrup, maple syrup, brown-rice syrup, molasses, evaporated cane
juice, cane juice, fruit-juice concentrate, corn sweetener.

ACKNOWLEDGMENTS

Any journalistic project that's been in the works as long as this one is bound to have required the help, faith, talent, and patience of so many sources, editors, researchers, and friends that enumerating them all is an effectively impossible job. To all of them, though, I am exceedingly grateful.

For this book alone, I'd like to thank Dave Dixon, Petro Dobromylskyj (aka "hyperlipid"), Mike Eades, Stephan Guyenet, Kevin Hall, Larry Istrail, Robert Kaplan, Adam Kosloff, Rick Lindquist, Ellen Rogers, Gary Sides, Frank Spence, Nassim Taleb, Clifford Taubes, Sonya Treyo, Mary Vernon, and Eric Westman, all of whom took the time to read a draft of this book and give me their thoughtful critiques and ideas for how to improve it. Ellen Rogers was also kind enough to do the illustrations and help me bring a little clarity to the subject of fat metabolism; Bob Kaplan was generous with his time and his impressive skills as a researcher. I'm grateful to Mary Dan and Mike Eades, Stephen Phinney, Mary Vernon, Eric Westman, and Jay Wortman for taking the time to discuss what they've learned about treating patients with carbohydrate-restricted diets. I'd like to thank Duane Storey for his gracious help with my website, and Ulrike Gonder for her research in Germany.

I'd like to thank Jimmy Moore for being, well, Jimmy Moore.

Thanks, once again, to Hugo Lindgren and Adam Moss; to Adam Fisher for his editing of my article "The Scientist and the Stairmaster" in *New York* magazine; and Rebecca Milzoff for her fact-checking.

At Knopf, my peerless editor Jon Segal first made this book happen and then made it work. Thanks go to Kyle McCarthy and

Acknowledgments

Joey McGarvey for their expert and endlessly cheerful assistance. My agent, Kris Dahl, at ICM continues to make me grateful for her friendship and her support.

My wife, Sloane Tanen, makes this possible (and tosses enough hibernating African llamas into the mix to keep it amusing). Our sons, Harry and Nick, make it worth the effort.

SOURCES

The list below includes relevant sources for each chapter and, in some cases, academic review articles or books that provide reasonably balanced analyses of the science. As I suggested in the Author's Note, those who are serious about deconstructing my conclusions in this book (or challenging them) and the history of the relevant nutritional issues should refer to *Good Calories, Bad Calories* for the logic, the evidence, and the more detailed annotations.

Introduction: The Original Sin

Bruch, H. 1957. *The Importance of Overweight.* New York: W. W. Norton.

Gladwell, M. 1998. "The Pima Paradox." *The New Yorker.* Feb 2.

Pollan, M. 2008. *In Defense of Food.* New York: Penguin Press.

Renold, A. E., and G. F. Cahill, Jr., eds. 1965. *Handbook of Physiology, Section 5, Adipose Tissue.* Washington, D.C.: American Physiological Society.

Chapter 1: Why Were They Fat?

Arteaga, A. 1974. "The Nutritional Status of Latin American Adults." In *Nutrition and Agricultural Development*, ed. N. S. Scrimshaw and B. Moises, pp. 67–76. New York: Plenum Press.

Brownell, K. D., and G. B. Horgen. 2004. *Food Fight: The Inside Story of the Food Industry, America's Obesity Crisis, and What We Can Do About It.* New York: McGraw-Hill.

Caballero, B. 2005. "A Nutrition Paradox—Underweight and Obesity in Developing Countries." *New England Journal of Medicine.* Apr 14;352(15): 1514–16.

Dobyns, H. F. 1989. *The Pima-Maricopa.* New York: Chelsea House.

Goldblatt, P. B., M. E. Moore, and A. J. Stunkard. 1965. "Social Factors in Obesity." *Journal of the American Medical Association.* Jun 21;192:1039–44.

Grant, F. W., and D. Groom. 1959. "A Dietary Study Among a Group of Southern Negroes." *Journal of the American Dietetics Association.* Sep;35:910–18.

Haddock, D. R. 1969. "Obesity in Medical Out-Patients in Accra." *Ghana Medical Journal.* Dec:251–54.

Helstosky, C. F. 2004. *Garlic and Oil: Food and Politics in Italy.* Oxford, U.K.: Berg Publishers.

Hrdlička, A. 1908. *Physiological and Medical Observations Among the Indians of Southwestern United States and Northern Mexico.* Washington, D.C.: U.S. Government Printing Office.

———. 1906. "Notes on the Pima of Arizona." *American Anthropologist.* Jan–Mar;8(1):39–46.

Interdepartmental Commission on Nutrition for National Defense. 1962. *Nutrition Survey in the West Indies.* Washington, D.C.: U.S. Government Printing Office.

Johnson, T. O. 1970. "Prevalence of Overweight and Obesity Among Adult Subjects of an Urban African Population Sample." *British Journal of Preventive & Social Medicine.* 24;105–9.

Keys, A. 1983. "From Naples to Seven Countries—A Sentimental Journey." *Progress in Biochemical Pharmacology.* 19:1–30.

Kraus, B. R. 1954. *Indian Health in Arizona: A Study of Health Conditions Among Central and Southern Arizona Indians.* Tucson: University of Arizona Press.

Lewis, N. 1978. *Naples '44.* New York: Pantheon.

McCarthy C. 1966. "Dietary and Activity Patterns of Obese Women in Trinidad." *Journal of the American Dietetics Association.* Jan;48:33–37.

Nestle, M. 2003. "The Ironic Politics of Obesity." *Science.* Feb 7;269(5608):781.

Osancova, K. 1975. "Trends of Dietary Intake and Prevalence of Obesity in Czechoslovakia." In *Recent Advances in Obesity Research: I,* ed. A. N. Howard, pp. 42–50. Westport, Conn.: Technomic Publishing.

Prior, I. A. 1971. "The Price of Civilization." *Nutrition Today.* Jul–Aug:2–11.

Reichley, K. B., W. H. Mueller, C. L. Hanis, et al. 1987. "Centralized Obesity and Cardiovascular Disease Risk in Mexican Americans." *American Journal of Epidemiology.* Mar;125(3):373–86.

Richards, R., and M. deCasseres. 1974. "The Problem of Obesity in Developing Countries: Its Prevalence and Morbidity." In *Obesity,* ed. W. L. Burland, P. D. Samuel, and J. Yudkin, pp. 74–84. New York: Churchill Livingstone.

Russell, F. 1975. *The Pima Indians.* Tuscon: University of Arizona Press. [Originally published 1908.]

Sources

Seftel, H. C., K. J. Keeley, A. R. Walker, J. J. Theron, and D. Delange. 1965. "Coronary Heart Disease in Aged South African Bantu." *Geriatrics.* Mar;20:194–205.

Slome, C., B. Gampel, J. H. Abramson, and N. Scotch. 1960. "Weight, Height and Skinfold Thickness of Zulu Adults in Durban." *South African Medical Journal.* Jun 11;34:505–9.

Stein, J. H., K. M. West, J. M. Robey, D. F. Tirador, and G. W. McDonald. 1965. "The High Prevalence of Abnormal Glucose Tolerance in the Cherokee Indians of North Carolina." *Archives of Internal Medicine.* Dec;116(6): 842–45.

Stene, J. A., and I. L. Roberts. 1928. "A Nutrition Study on an Indian Reservation." *Journal of the American Dietetics Association.* Mar;3(4):215–22.

Tulloch, J. A. 1962. *Diabetes Mellitus in the Tropics.* London: Livingstone.

Valente, S., A. Arteaga, and J. Santa Maria. 1964. "Obesity in a Developing Country." In *Proceedings of the Sixth International Congress of Nutrition,* ed. C. F. Mills and R. Passmore, p. 555. Edinburgh: Livingstone.

Walker, A. R. 1964. "Overweight and Hypertension in Emerging Populations." *American Heart Journal.* Nov;68(5):581–85.

West, K. M. 1981. "North American Indians." In *Western Diseases,* ed. H. C. Trowell and D. P. Burkitt, pp. 129–37. London: Edward Arnold.

Chapter 2: The Elusive Benefits of Undereating

Dansinger, M. L., A. Tatsioni, W. B. Wong, M. Chung, and E. M. Balk. 2007. "Meta-Analysis: The Effect of Dietary Counseling for Weight Loss." *The Archives of Internal Medicine.* Jul 3;147(1):41–50.

Howard, B. V., J. E. Manson, M. L. Stefanick, et al. 2006. "Low-Fat Dietary Pattern and Weight Change over 7 Years: The Women's Health Initiative Dietary Modification Trial." *Journal of the American Medical Association.* Jan 4;295(1):39–49.

Maratos-Flier, E., and J. S. Flier. 2005. "Obesity." In *Joslin's Diabetes Mellitus.* 14th ed., ed. C. R. Kahn, G. C. Weir, G. L. King, A. C. Moses, R. J. Smith, and A. M. Jacobson, pp. 533–45. Media, Pa.: Lippincott, Williams & Wilkins.

Palgi, A., J. L. Read, I. Greenberg, M. A. Hoefer, R. R. Bistrian, and G. L. Blackburn. 1985. "Multidisciplinary Treatment of Obesity with a Protein-Sparing Modified Fast: Results in 668 Outpatients." *American Journal of Public Health.* Oct;75(10):1190–94.

Sources

Pollan, M. 2007. "Unhappy Meals." *New York Times.* Jan 28.

Sacks, G. A., G. A. Bray, V. J. Carey, et al. 2009. "Comparison of Weight-Loss Diets with Different Compositions of Fat, Protein, and Carbohydrates." *New England Journal of Medicine.* Feb 26;360(9):859–73.

Stunkard, A., and M. McClaren-Hume. 1959. "The Results of Treatment for Obesity: A Review of the Literature and a Report of a Series." *Archives of Internal Medicine.* Jan;103(1):79–85.

Van Gaal, L. F. 1998. "Dietary Treatment of Obesity." In *Handbook of Obesity,* ed. G. A. Bray, C. Bouchard, and W.P.T. James, pp. 875–90. New York: Marcel Dekker.

Chapter 3: The Elusive Benefits of Exercise

Bennett, W., and J. Gurin. 1982. *The Dieter's Dilemma: Eating Less and Weighing More.* New York: Basic Books.

Bray, G. A. 1979. *Obesity in America.* Public Health Service, National Institutes of Health, NIH Publication No. 79–359.

Cohn, V. 1980. "A Passion to Keep Fit: 100 Million Americans Exercising." *Washington Post.* Aug 31:A1.

Elia, M. 1992. "Organ and Tissue Contribution to Metabolic Rate." In *Energy Metabolism,* ed. J. M. Kinney and H. N. Tucker, pp. 61–79. New York: Raven Press.

Fogelholm, M., and K. Kukkonen-Harjula. 2000. "Does Physical Activity Prevent Weight Gain—a Systematic Review." *Obesity Reviews.* Oct;1(2):95–111.

Gilmore, C. P. 1977. "Taking Exercise to Heart." *New York Times.* Mar 27:211.

Haskell, W. L., I. M. Lee, R. R. Pate, et al. 2007. "Physical Activity and Public Health: Updated Recommendation for Adults from the American College of Sports Medicine and the American Heart Association." *Circulation.* Aug 28;116(9):1081–93.

Janssen, G. M., C. J. Graef, and W. H. Saris. 1989. "Food Intake and Body Composition in Novice Athletes During a Training Period to Run a Marathon." *International Journal of Sports Medicine.* May;10(Suppl 1):S17–S21.

Kolata, G. 2004. *Ultimate Fitness.* New York: Picador.

Mayer J. 1968. *Overweight: Causes, Cost, and Control.* Englewood Cliffs, N.J.: Prentice-Hall.

Mayer, J., and F. J. Stare. 1953. "Exercise and Weight Control." *Journal of the American Dietetic Association.* Apr;29(4):340–43.

Sources

Mayer, J., N. B. Marshall, J. J. Vitale, J. H. Christensen, M. B. Mashayekhi, and F. J. Stare. 1954. "Exercise, Food Intake and Body Weight in Normal Rats and Genetically Obese Adult Mice." *American Journal of Physiology.* Jun;177(3):544–48.

Mayer, J., P. Roy, and K. P. Mitra. 1956. "Relation Between Caloric Intake, Body Weight, and Physical Work: Studies in an Industrial Male Population in West Bengal." *American Journal of Clinical Nutrition.* Mar–Apr;4(2):169–75.

Newburgh, L. H. 1942. "Obesity." *Archives of Internal Medicine.* Dec;70: 1033–96.

Rony, H. R. 1940. *Obesity and Leanness.* Philadelphia: Lea & Febiger.

Segal, K. R., and F. X. Pi-Sunyer. 1989. "Exercise and Obesity." *Medical Clinics of North America.* Jan;73(1):217–36.

Stern, J. S., and P. Lowney. 1986. "Obesity: The Role of Physical Activity." In *Handbook of Eating Disorders*, ed. K. D Brownell and J. P. Foreyt, pp. 145–58. New York: Basic Books.

Wilder, R. M. 1933. "The Treatment of Obesity." *International Clinics.* 4:1–21.

Williams, P. T., and P. D. Wood. 2006. "The Effects of Changing Exercise Levels on Weight and Age-Related Weight Gain." *International Journal of Obesity.* Mar;30(3):543–51.

Chapter 4: The Significance of Twenty Calories a Day

Du Bois, E. F. 1936. *Basal Metabolism in Health and Disease.* 2nd ed. Philadelphia: Lea & Febiger.

Chapter 5: Why Me? Why There? Why Then?

Bauer, J. 1941. "Obesity: Its Pathogenesis, Etiology and Treatment." *Archives of Internal Medicine.* May;67(5):968–94.

———. 1940. "Observations on Obese Children." *Archives of Pediatrics.* 57: 631–40.

Bergmann, G. von, and F. Stroebe. 1927. "Die Fettsucht." In *Handbuch der Biochemie des Menschen und der Tiere*, ed. C. Oppenheimer, pp. 562–98. Jena, Germany: Verlag von Gustav Fischer.

Grafe, E. 1933. *Metabolic Diseases and Their Treatment.* Trans. M. G. Boise. Philadelphia: Lea & Febiger.

Jones, E. 1956. "Progressive Lipodystrophy." *British Medical Journal.* Feb 11;4962(1):313–19.

Sources

Moreno, S., C. Miralles, E. Negredo, et al. 2009. "Disorders of Body Fat Distribution in HIV-1-Infected Patients." *AIDS Review.* Jul–Sep;11(3):126–34.

Silver, S., and J. Bauer. 1931. "Obesity, Constitutional or Endocrine?" *American Journal of Medical Science.* 181:769–77.

Chapter 6: Thermodynamics for Dummies, Part 1

Mayer, J. 1954. "Multiple Causative Factors in Obesity." In *Fat Metabolism*, ed. V. A. Najjar, pp. 22–43. Baltimore: Johns Hopkins University Press.

National Institutes of Health. 1998. *Clinical Guidelines on the Identification, Evaluation, and Treatment of Overweight and Obesity in Adults: The Evidence Report.* NIH Publication No. 98–4083.

Noorden, C. von. 1907. "Obesity." Trans. D. Spence. In *The Pathology of Metabolism*, vol. 3 of *Metabolism and Practical Medicine*, ed. C. von Noorden and I. W. Hall, pp. 693–715. Chicago: W. Keener.

Chapter 7: Thermodynamics for Dummies, Part 2

Flier, J. S., and E. Maratos-Flier. 2007. "What Fuels Fat." *Scientific American.* Sep;297(3):72–81.

Chapter 8: Head Cases

Astwood, E. B. 1962. "The Heritage of Corpulence." *Endocrinology.* Aug;71: 337–41.

Bauer, J. 1947. *Constitution and Disease: Applied Constitutional Pathology.* New York: Grune & Stratton.

Lustig, R. 2006. "Childhood Obesity: Behavioral Aberration or Biochemical Drive? Reinterpreting the First Law of Thermodynamics." *Nature Clinical Practice. Endocrinology & Metabolism.* Aug;2(8):447–58.

Newburgh, L. H. 1931. "The Cause of Obesity." *Journal of the American Medical Association.* Dec 5;97(23):1659–63.

Rony, H. R. 1940. *Obesity and Leanness.* Philadelphia: Lea & Febiger.

Sontag, S. 1990. *Illness as Metaphor and AIDS and Its Metaphors.* New York: Picador.

Chapter 9: The Laws of Adiposity

Bergmann, G. von, and F. Stroebe. 1927. "Die Fettsucht." In *Handbuch der Biochemie des Menschen und der Tiere*, ed. C. Oppenheimer, pp. 562–98. Jena, Germany: Verlag von Gustav Fischer.

Sources

Björntorp, P. 1997. "Hormonal Control of Regional Fat Distribution." *Human Reproduction*. Oct;12 (Suppl 1):21–25.

Brooks, C. M. 1946. "The Relative Importance of Changes in Activity in the Development of Experimentally Produced Obesity in the Rat." *American Journal of Physiology*. Dec;147:708–16.

Greenwood, M. R., M. Cleary, L. Steingrimsdottir, and J. R. Vaselli. 1981. "Adipose Tissue Metabolism and Genetic Obesity." In *Recent Advances in Obesity Research: III*, ed. P. Björntorp, M. Cairella, and A. N. Howard, pp. 75–79. London: John Libbey.

Hetherington, A. W., and S. W. Ranson. 1942. "The Spontaneous Activity and Food Intake of Rats with Hypothalamic Lesions." *American Journal of Physiology*. Jun;136(4):609–17.

Kronenberg, H. M., S. Melmed, K. S. Polonsky, and P. R. Larsen. 2008. *Williams Textbook of Endocrinology*. Philadelphia: Saunders.

Mayer, J. 1968. *Overweight: Causes, Cost, and Control*. Englewood Cliffs, N.J.: Prentice-Hall.

Mrosovsky, N. 1976. "Lipid Programmes and Life Strategies in Hibernators." *American Zoologist*. 16:685–97.

Rebuffé-Scrive, M. 1987. "Regional Adipose Tissue Metabolism in Women During and After Reproductive Life and in Men." In *Recent Advances in Obesity Research: V*, ed. E. M. Berry, S. H. Blondheim, H. E. Eliahou, and E. Shafrir, pp. 82–91. London: John Libbey.

Wade, G. N., and J. E. Schneider. 1992. "Metabolic Fuels and Reproduction in Female Mammals." *Neuroscience and Behavioral Reviews*. Summer;16(2):235–72.

Chapter 10: A Historical Digression on "Lipophilia"

Astwood, E. B. 1962. "The Heritage of Corpulence." *Endocrinology*. Aug;71: 337–41.

Bergmann, G. von, and F. Stroebe. 1927. "Die Fettsucht." In *Handbuch der Biochemie des Menschen und der Tiere*, ed. C. Oppenheimer, pp. 562–98. Jena, Germany: Verlag von Gustav Fischer.

Bruch, H. 1973. *Eating Disorders: Obesity, Anorexia Nervosa, and the Person Within*. New York: Basic Books.

Mayer, J. 1968. *Overweight: Causes, Cost, and Control*. Englewood Cliffs, N.J.: Prentice-Hall.

Rony, H. R. 1940. *Obesity and Leanness*. Philadelphia: Lea & Febiger.

Sources

Silver, S., and J. Bauer. 1931. "Obesity, Constitutional or Endocrine?" *American Journal of Medical Science*. 181:769–77.

Wilder, R. M., and W. L. Wilbur. 1938. "Diseases of Metabolism and Nutrition." *Archives of Internal Medicine*. Feb;61:297–65.

Chapter 11: A Primer on the Regulation of Fat

Action to Control Cardiovascular Risk in Diabetes Study Group. 2008. "Effects of Intensive Glucose Lowering in Type 2 Diabetes." *New England Journal of Medicine*. June 12;358(24):2545–59.

Berson, S. A., and R. S. Yalow. 1970. "Insulin 'Antagonists' and Insulin Resistance." In *Diabetes Mellitus: Theory and Practice*, ed. M. Ellenberg and H. Rifkin, pp. 388–423. New York: McGraw-Hill.

———. 1965. "Some Current Controversies in Diabetes Research." *Diabetes*. Sep;14:549–72.

Fielding, B. A., and K. N. Frayn. 1998. "Lipoprotein Lipase and the Disposition of Dietary Fatty Acids." *British Journal of Nutrition*. Dec;80(6):495–502.

Frayn, K. N., F. Karpe, B. A. Fielding, I. A. Macdonald, and S. W. Coppack. 2003. "Integrative Physiology of Human Adipose Tissue." *International Journal of Obesity*. Aug;27(8):875–88.

Friedman, M. I., and E. M. Stricker. 1976. "The Physiological Psychology of Hunger: A Physiological Perspective." *Psychological Review*. Nov;83(6): 409–31.

Le Magnen, J. 1984. "Is Regulation of Body Weight Elucidated?" *Neuroscience & Biobehavioral Review*. Winter;8(4):515–22.

Newsholme, E. A., and C. Start. 1973. *Regulation in Metabolism*. New York: John Wiley.

Nussey, S. S., and S. A. Whitehead. 2001. *Endocrinology: An Integrated Approach*. London: Taylor & Francis.

Renold, A. E., O. B. Crofford, W. Stauffacher, and B. Jeanreaud. 1965. "Hormonal Control of Adipose Tissue Metabolism: With Special Reference to the Effects of Insulin." *Diabetologia*. Aug;1(1):4–12.

Rosenzweig, J. L. 1994. "Principles of Insulin Therapy." In *Joslin's Diabetes Mellitus*, 13th ed., ed. C. R. Kahn and G. C. Weir, pp. 460–88. Media, Pa.: Lippincott, Williams & Wilkins.

Wertheimer, E., and R. Shapiro. 1948. "The Physiology of Adipose Tissue." *Physiological Reviews*. Oct;28:451–64.

Wood, P. A. 2006. *How Fat Works*. Cambridge, Mass.: Harvard University Press.

Sources

Chapter 12: Why I Get Fat and You Don't (or Vice Versa)

Bluher, M., B. B. Kahn, and C. R. Kahn. 2003. "Extended Longevity in Mice Lacking the Insulin Receptor in Adipose Tissue." *Science.* Jan 24;299 (5606):572–74.

Dabalea, D. 2007. "The Predisposition to Obesity and Diabetes in Offspring of Diabetic Mothers." *Diabetes Care.* July;30(Suppl 2):S169–S174.

Dabelea, D., W. C. Knowler, and D. J. Pettitt. 2000. "Effect of Diabetes in Pregnancy on Offspring: Follow-Up Research in the Pima Indians." *Journal of Maternal-Fetal Medicine.* Jan–Feb;9(1):83–88.

DeFronzo, R. A. 1997. "Insulin Resistance: A Multifaceted Syndrome Responsible for NIDDM, Obesity, Hypertension, Dyslipidaemia and Atherosclerosis." *Netherlands Journal of Medicine.* May;50(5):191–97.

Kim, J., K. E. Peterson, K. S. Scanlon, et al. 2006. "Trends in Overweight from 1980 through 2001 Among Preschool-Aged Children Enrolled in a Health Maintenance Organization." *Obesity.* July;14(7):1107–12.

McGarry, D. J. 1992. "What If Minkowski Had Been Ageusic? An Alternative Angle on Diabetes." *Science.* Oct 30;258(5083):766–770.

McGowan, C. A., and F. M. McAuliffe. 2010. "The Influence of Maternal Glycaemia and Dietary Glycaemic Index on Pregnancy Outcome in Healthy Mothers." *British Journal of Nutrition.* Mar 23:1–7.

Metzger, B. E. 2007. "Long-Term Outcomes in Mothers Diagnosed with Gestational Diabetes Mellitus and Their Offspring." *Clinical Obstetrics and Gynecology.* Dec;50(4):972–79.

Neel, J. V. 1982. "The Thrifty Genotype Revisited." In *The Genetics of Diabetes Mellitus.* ed. J. Köbberling and R. Tattersall, pp. 283–93. New York: Academic Press.

Chapter 13: What We Can Do

Jenkins, D. J., C. W. Kendall, L. S. Augustin, et al. 2002. "Glycemic Index: Overview of Implications in Health and Disease." *American Journal of Clinical Nutrition.* Jul;76(1):266S–73S.

Johnson, R. K., L. J. Appel, M. Brands, et al. 2009. "Dietary Sugars Intake and Cardiovascular Health: A Scientific Statement from the American Heart Association." *Circulation.* Sep 15;120(11):1011–20.

Mayes, P. A. 1993. "Intermediary Metabolism of Fructose." *American Journal of Clinical Nutrition.* Nov;58(Suppl 5):754S–65S.

Stanhope, K. L., and P. J. Havel. 2008. "Endocrine and Metabolic Effects of Consuming Beverages Sweetened with Fructose, Glucose, Sucrose, or

High-Fructose Corn Syrup." *American Journal of Clinical Nutrition.* Dec;88(6):1733S–37S.

Stanhope, K. L., J. M. Schwarz, N. L. Keim, et al. 2009. "Consuming Fructose-Sweetened, Not Glucose-Sweetened, Beverages Increases Visceral Adiposity and Lipids and Decreases Insulin Sensitivity in Overweight/Obese Humans." *Journal of Clinical Investigation.* May 1;119(5):1322–34.

Chapter 14: Injustice Collecting

Avena, N. M., P. Rava, and B. G. Hoebel. 2008. "Evidence for Sugar Addiction: Behavioral and Neurochemical Effects of Intermittent, Excessive Sugar Intake." *Neuroscience & Biobehavioral Reviews.* 32(1):20–39.

Le Magnen, J. 1985. *Hunger.* Cambridge: Cambridge University Press.

Chapter 15: Why Diets Succeed and Fail

Gardner, C. D., A. Kiazand, S. Alhassan, et al. 2007. "Comparison of the Atkins, Zone, Ornish, and LEARN Diets for Change in Weight and Related Risk Factors Among Overweight Premenopausal Women: The A TO Z Weight Loss Study, a Randomized Trial." *Journal of the American Medical Association.* Mar 7;297(9):969–77.

Ornish, D. 1996. "Very Low-Fat Diets for Coronary Heart Disease: Perhaps, but Which One?—Reply." *Jounal of the American Medical Association.* May 8;275(18):1403.

Shai, I., D. Schwarzfuchs, Y. Henkin, et al. 2008. "Weight Loss with a Low-Carbohydrate, Mediterranean, or Low-Fat Diet." *New England Journal of Medicine.* Jul 17;359(3):229–41.

Chapter 16: A Historical Digression on the Fattening Carbohydrate

Anon. 1973. "A Critique of Low-Carbohydrate Ketogenic Weight Reduction Regimens: A Review of 'Dr. Atkins' Diet Revolution.' " *Journal of the American Medical Association.* Jun 4;224(10):1415–19.

Anon. 1995. *An Eating Plan for Healthy Americans: The American Heart Association Diet.* Dallas: American Heart Association.

Apfelbaum, M., ed. 1973. *Regulation de l'équilibre énergetique chez l'homme.* [*Energy Balance in Man.*] Paris: Masson et Cie.

Banting, W. 2005. *Letter on Corpulence, Addressed to the Public.* 4th ed. London: Harrison. Republished New York: Cosimo Publishing. [Originally published in 1864.]

Sources

Borders, W. 1965. "New Diet Decried by Nutritionists; Dangers Are Seen in Low Carbohydrate Intake." *New York Times*. July 7:16.

Bray, G. A., ed. 1976. *Obesity in Perspective*. DHEW Pub No. (NIH) 76–852. Washington, D.C.: U.S. Government Printing Office.

Brillat-Savarin, J. A. 1986. *The Physiology of Taste*. Trans. M. F. K. Fisher. San Francisco: North Point Press. [Originally published in 1825.]

Bruch, H. 1957. *The Importance of Overweight*. New York: W. W. Norton.

Burland, W. L., P. D. Samuel, and J. Yudkin, eds. 1974. *Obesity*. New York: Churchill Livingstone.

Cutting, W. C. 1943. "The Treatment of Obesity." *Journal of Clinical Endocrinology*. Feb;3(2):85–88.

Dancel, J. F. 1864. *Obesity, or Excessive Corpulence: The Various Causes and the Rational Means of Cure*. Trans. M. Barrett. Toronto: W. C. Chewett.

Davidson, S., and R. Passmore. 1963. *Human Nutrition and Dietetics*. 2nd ed. Edinburgh: E.&S. Livingstone.

French, J. M. 1907. *A Text-Book of the Practice of Medicine, for Students and Practitioners*. 3rd, rev. ed. New York: William Wood.

Gardiner-Hill, H. 1925. "The Treatment of Obesity." *Lancet*. Nov 14;206(5333): 1034–35.

Gordon, E. S., M. Goldberg, and G. J. Chosy. 1963. "A New Concept in the Treatment of Obesity." *Journal of the American Medical Association*. Oct 5;186:50–60.

Greene, R., ed. 1951. *The Practice of Endocrinology*. Philadelphia: J. B. Lippincott.

Hanssen, P. 1936. "Treatment of Obesity by a Diet Relatively Poor in Carbohydrates." *Acta Medica Scandinavica*. 88:97–106.

Harvey, W. 1872. *On Corpulence in Relation to Disease: With Some Remarks on Diet*. London: Henry Renshaw.

Hastings, M. 2008. *Retribution: The Battle for Japan, 1944–45*. New York: Alfred A. Knopf.

Krehl, W. A., A. Lopez, E. I. Good, and R. E. Hodges. 1967. "Some Metabolic Changes Induced by Low Carbohydrate Diets." *American Journal of Clinical Nutrition*. Feb;20(2):139–48.

LaRosa, J. C., A. Gordon, R. Muesing, and D. R. Rosing. 1980. "Effects of High-Protein, Low-Carbohydrate Dieting on Plasma Lipoproteins and Body Weight." *Journal of the American Dietetics Association*. Sep;77(3):264–70.

Sources

Leith, W. 1961. "Experiences with the Pennington Diet in the Management of Obesity." *Canadian Medical Association Journal.* Jun 24;84:1411–14.

McLean Baird, I., and A. N. Howard, eds. 1969. *Obesity: Medical and Scientific Aspects.* London: Livingstone.

Milch, L. J., W. J. Walker, and N. Weiner. 1957. "Differential Effect of Dietary Fat and Weight Reduction on Serum Levels of Beta-Lipoproteins." *Circulation.* Jan;15(1):31–34.

Ohlson, M. A., W. D. Brewer, D. Kereluk, A. Wagoner, and D. C. Cederquist. 1955. "Weight Control Through Nutritionally Adequate Diets." In *Weight Control: A Collection of Papers Presented at the Weight Control Colloquium,* ed. E. S. Eppright, P. Swanson, and C. A. Iverson, pp. 170–87. Ames: Iowa State College Press.

Osler, W. 1901. *The Principles and Practice of Medicine.* New York: D. Appleton.

Palmgren, B., and B. Sjövall. 1957. "Studier Rörande Fetma: IV, Forsook Med Pennington-Diet." *Nordisk Medicin.* 28(iii):457–58.

Passmore, R., and Y. E. Swindells. 1963. "Observations on the Respiratory Quotients and Weight Gain of Man After Eating Large Quantities of Carbohydrate." *British Journal of Nutrition.* 17:331–39.

Pena, L., M. Pena, J. Gonzalez, and A. Claro. 1979. "A Comparative Study of Two Diets in the Treatment of Primary Exogenous Obesity in Children." *Acta Paediatrica Academiae Scientiarum Hungaricae.* 20(1):99–103.

Pennington, A. W. 1954. "Treatment of Obesity: Developments of the Past 150 Years." *American Journal of Digestive Diseases.* Mar;21(3):65–69.

——. 1953. "A Reorientation on Obesity." *New England Journal of Medicine.* Jun 4;248(23):959–64.

——. 1951. "Caloric Requirements of the Obese." *Industrial Medicine & Surgery.* Jun;20(6):267–71.

——. 1951. "The Use of Fat in a Weight Reducing Diet." *Delaware State Medical Journal.* Apr;23(4):79–86.

——. 1949. "Obesity in Industry—The Problem and Its Solution." *Industrial Medicine.* June: 259–60.

Reader, G., R. Melchionna, L. E. Hinkle, et al. 1952. "Treatment of Obesity." *American Journal of Medicine.* 13(4):478–86.

Rilliet, B. 1954. "Treatment of Obesity by a Low-calorie Diet: Hanssen-Boller-Pennington Diet." *Praxis.* Sep 9;43(36):761–63.

Silverstone, J. T., and F. Lockhead. 1963. "The Value of a 'Low Carbohydrate' Diet in Obese Diabetics." *Metabolism.* Aug;12(8):710–13.

Sources

Spock, B. 1985. *Baby and Child Care.* 5th ed. New York: Pocket Books.

———. 1976. *Baby and Child Care.* 4th ed. New York: Hawthorne Books.

———. 1968. *Baby and Child Care.* 3rd ed. New York: Meredith Press.

———. 1957. *The Common Sense Book of Baby and Child Care.* 2nd ed. New York: Duell, Sloan and Pearce.

———. 1946. *The Common Sense Book of Baby and Child Care.* New York: Duell, Sloan and Pearce.

Spock, B., and M. B. Rothenberg. 1992. *Dr. Spock's Baby and Child Care.* 6th ed. New York: E. P. Dutton.

Steiner, M. M. 1950. "The Management of Obesity in Childhood." *Medical Clinics of North America.* Jan;34(1):223–34.

Tanner, T. H. 1869. *The Practice of Medicine.* 6th ed. London: Henry Renshaw.

Williams, R. H., W. H. Daughaday, W. F. Rogers, S. P. Asper, and B. T. Towery. 1948. "Obesity and Its Treatment, with Particular Reference to the Use of Anorexigenic Compounds." *Annals of Internal Medicine.* 29(3):510–32.

Wilson, N. L., ed. 1969. *Obesity.* Philadelphia: F. A. Davis.

Young, C. M. 1976. "Dietary Treatment of Obesity." In *Obesity in Perspective,* ed. G. A. Bray, pp. 361–66. DHEW Pub No. (NIH) 76–852.

Chapter 17: Meat or Plants?

Anon. 1899. "The Month." *Practitioner.* 62:369. Cited in R. N. Proctor, *Cancer Wars.* New York: Basic Books: 1995.

Burkitt, D. P., and H. C. Trowell, eds. 1975. *Refined Carbohydrate Foods and Disease: Some Implications of Dietary Fibre.* New York: Academic Press.

Cleave, T. L., and G. D. Campbell. 1966. *Diabetes, Coronary Thrombosis and the Saccharine Disease.* Bristol, U.K.: John Wright & Sons.

Cordain, L., J. B. Miller, S. B. Eaton, N. Mann, S. H. Holt, and J. D. Speth. 2000. "Plant-Animal Subsistence Ratios and Macronutrient Energy Estimations in Worldwide Hunter-Gatherer Diets." *American Journal of Clinical Nutrition.* Mar;71(3):682–92.

Doll, R., and R. Peto. 1981. "The Causes of Cancer: Quantitative Estimates of Avoidable Risks of Cancer in the United States Today." *Journal of the National Cancer Institute.* Jun;66(6):1191–1308.

Donaldson, B. F. 1962. *Strong Medicine.* Garden City, N.Y.: Doubleday.

Higginson, J. 1997. "From Geographical Pathology to Environmental Carcinogenesis: A Historical Reminiscence." *Cancer Letters.* 117:133–42.

Sources

Levin, I. 1910. "Cancer Among the North American Indians and Its Bearing Upon the Ethnological Distribution of Disease." *Zeitschrift für Krebfoschung.* Oct;9(3):422–35.

Pollan, M. 2008. *In Defense of Food.* New York: Penguin Press.

Rose, G. 1985. "Sick Individuals and Sick Populations." *International Journal of Epidemiology.* Mar;14(1);32–38.

——. 1981. "Strategy of Prevention: Lessons from Cardiovascular Disease." *British Medical Journal.* Jun 6;282(6279):1847–51.

Trowell, H. C., and D. P. Burkitt, eds. 1981. *Western Diseases: Their Emergence and Prevention.* London: Edward Arnold.

Chapter 18: The Nature of a Healthy Diet

Basu, T. K., and C. J. Schlorah. 1982. *Vitamin C in Health and Disease.* Westport, Conn.: Avi Publishing.

Bode, A. M. 1997. "Metabolism of Vitamin C in Health and Disease." *Advanced Pharmacology.* 38:21–47.

Bravata, D. M., L. Sanders, J. Huang, et al. 2003. "Efficacy and Safety of Low-Carbohydrate Diets: A Systematic Review." *Journal of the American Medical Association.* Apr 9;289(14):1837–50.

Brehm, B. J., R. J. Seeley, S. R. Daniels, and D. A. D'Alessio. 2003. "A Randomized Trial Comparing a Very Low Carbohydrate Diet and a Calorie-Restricted Low Fat Diet on Body Weight and Cardiovascular Risk Factors in Healthy Women." *Journal of Clinical Endocrinology and Metabolism.* Apr;88(4):1617–23.

Calle, E. E., and R. Kaaks. 2004. "Overweight, Obesity and Cancer: Epidemiological Evidence and Proposed Mechanisms." *Nature Reviews Cancer.* Aug;4(8):579–91.

Cholesterol Education Program (NCEP) Expert Panel on Detection, Evaluation, and Treatment of High Blood Cholesterol in Adults. 2002. "(Adult Treatment Panel III) Final report." *Circulation.* Dec 17;106(25):3143–3421.

Cox, B. D., M. J. Whichelow, W. J. Butterfield, and P. Nicholas. 1974. "Peripheral Vitamin C Metabolism in Diabetics and Non-Diabetics: Effect of Intra-Arterial Insulin." *Clinical Sciences & Molecular Medicine.* Jul;47(1):63–72.

Cunningham, J. J. 1998. "The Glucose/Insulin System and Vitamin C: Implications in Insulin-Dependent Diabetes Mellitus." *Journal of the American College of Nutrition.* Apr;17(20):105–8.

——. 1988. "Altered Vitamin C Transport in Diabetes Mellitus." *Medical Hypotheses.* Aug;26(4):263–65.

Ernst, N. D., and R. I. Levy. 1984. "Diet and Cardiovascular Disease." In *Present Knowledge in Nutrition*, 5th ed., ed. R. E. Olson, H. P. Broquist, C. O. Chichester, et al., pp. 724–39. Washington, D.C.: Nutrition Foundation.

Ford, E. S., A. H. Mokdad, W. H. Giles, and D. W. Brown. 2003. "The Metabolic Syndrome and Antioxidant Concentrations: Findings from the Third National Health and Nutrition Examination Survey." *Diabetes*. Sep;52(9): 2346–52.

Foster, G. D., H. R. Wyatt, J. O. Hill, et al. 2010. "Weight and Metabolic Outcomes After 2 Years on a Low-Carbohydrate Versus Low-Fat Diet. A Randomized Trial." *Annals of Internal Medicine*. Aug 3;153(3):147–57.

———. 2003. "A Randomized Trial of a Low-Carbohydrate Diet for Obesity." *New England Journal of Medicine*. May 22;348(21):2082–90.

Freeman, J. M., E. H. Kossoff, and A. L. Hartman. 2007. "The Ketogenic Diet: One Decade Later." *Pediatrics*. Mar;119(3):535–43.

Gardner, C. D., A. Kiazand, S. Alhassan, et al. 2007. "Comparison of the Atkins, Zone, Ornish, and LEARN Diets for Change in Weight and Related Risk Factors Among Overweight Premenopausal Women: The A TO Z Weight Loss Study, a Randomized Trial." *Journal of the American Medical Association*. Mar 7;297(9):969–77.

Godsland, I. F. 2009. "Insulin Resistance and Hyperinsulinaemia in the Development and Progression of Cancer." *Clinical Science*. Nov 23;118(5):315–32.

Harris, M. 1985. *Good to Eat: Riddles of Food and Culture*. New York: Simon and Schuster.

Hession, M., C. Rolland, U. Kulkarni, A. Wise, and J. Broom. 2009. "Systematic Review of Randomized Controlled Trials of Low-Carbohydrate vs. Low-Fat/Low-Calorie Diets in the Management of Obesity and Its Comorbidities." *Obesity Reviews*. Jan;10(1):36–50.

Hooper, L., C. D. Summerbell, J. P. Higgins, et al. 2001. "Reduced or Modified Dietary Fat for Preventing Cardiovascular Disease." *Cochrane Database of Systematic Reviews*. (3):CD002137.

Howard, B. V., L. Van Horn, J. Hsia, et al. 2006. "Low-Fat Dietary Pattern and Risk of Cardiovascular Disease: The Women's Health Initiative Randomized Controlled Dietary Modification Trial." *Journal of the American Medical Association*. Feb 8;295(6):655–66.

Katan, M. B. 2009. "Weight-Loss Diets for the Prevention and Treatment of Obesity." *New England Journal of Medicine*. Feb 26;360(9):923–25.

Kuklina, E. V., P. W. Yoon, and N. L. Keenan. 2009. "Trends in High Levels of Low-Density Lipoprotein Cholesterol in the United States, 1999–2006." *Journal of the American Medical Association*. Nov 18;302(19):2104–10.

Sources

Luchsinger, J. A., and D. R. Gustafson. 2009. "Adiposity, Type 2 Diabetes, and Alzheimer's Disease." *Journal of Alzheimer's Disease.* Apr;16(4):693–704.

Maher, P. A., and D. R. Schubert. 2009. "Metabolic Links Between Diabetes and Alzheimer's Disease." *Expert Reviews of Neurotherapeutics.* Oct;111(2): 332–43.

Mavropoulos, J. C., W. B. Isaacs, S. V. Pizzo, and S. J. Freedland. 2006. "Is There a Role for a Low-Carbohydrate Ketogenic Diet in the Management of Prostate Cancer?" *Urology.* Jul;68(1):15–18.

Neal, E. G., and J. H. Cross. 2010. "Efficacy of Dietary Treatments for Epilepsy." *Journal of Human Nutrition and Dietetics.* Apr;23(2):113–19.

Packard, C. J. 2006. "Small Dense Low-Density Lipoprotein and Its Role as an Independent Predictor of Cardiovascular Disease." *Current Opinions in Lipidology.* Aug;17(4):412–17.

Sacks, G. A., G. A. Bray, V. J. Carey, et al. 2009. "Comparison of Weight-Loss Diets with Different Compositions of Fat, Protein, and Carbohydrates." *New England Journal of Medicine.* Feb 26;360(9):859–73.

Samaha, F. F., N. Iqubal, P. Seshadri, et al. 2003. "A Low-Carbohydrate as Compared with a Low-Fat Diet in Severe Obesity." *New England Journal of Medicine.* May 22;348(21):2074–81.

Seyfried, B. T., M. Klebish, J. Marsh, and P. Mukherjee. 2009. "Targeting Energy Metabolism in Brain Cancer Through Calorie Restriction and the Ketogenic Diet." *Journal of Cancer Research Therapy.* Sep;5(Suppl 1):S7–S15.

Shai, I., D. Schwarzfuchs, Y. Henkin, et al. 2008. "Weight Loss with a Low-Carbohydrate, Mediterranean, or Low-Fat Diet." *New England Journal of Medicine.* Jul 17;359(3):229–41.

Siri, P. M., and R. M. Krauss. 2005. "Influence of Dietary Carbohydrate and Fat on LDL and HDL Particle Distributions." *Current Atherosclerosis Reports.* Nov;7(6):455–59.

Skeaff, C. M., and J. Miller. 2009. "Dietary Fat and Coronary Heart Disease: Summary of Evidence from Prospective Cohort and Randomised Controlled Trials." *Annals of Nutrition & Metabolism.* 55(1–3):173–201.

Sondike, S. B., N. Copperman, and M. S. Jacobson. 2003. "Effects of a Low-Carbohydrate Diet on Weight Loss and Cardiovascular Risk Factor in Overweight Adolescents." *Journal of Pediatrics.* Mar;142(3):253–58.

Will, J. C., and T. Byers. 1996. "Does Diabetes Mellitus Increase the Requirement for Vitamin C?" *Nutrition Reviews.* Jul;54(7):193–202.

Wilson, P. W., and J. B. Meigs. 2008. "Cardiometabolic Risk: a Framingham Perspective." *International Journal of Obesity.* May;32(Suppl 2):S17–S20.

Sources

World Cancer Research Fund and American Institute for Cancer Research. 2007. *Food, Nutrition, Physical Activity and the Prevention of Cancer: a Global Perspective.* Washington, D.C.: American Institute for Cancer Research.

Yancy, W. S., Jr., M. K. Olsen, J. R. Guyton, R. P. Bakst, and E. C. Westman. 2004. "A Low-Carbohydrate, Ketogenic Diet Versus a Low-Fat Diet to Treat Obesity and Hyperlipidemia: A Randomized, Controlled Trial." *Annals of Internal Medicine.* May 18;140(10):769–77.

Chapter 19: Following Through

Allan, C. B., and W. Lutz. 2000. *Life Without Bread: How a Low-Carbohydrate Diet Can Save Your Life.* New York: McGraw-Hill.

Kemp, R. 1972. "The Over-All Picture of Obesity." *Practitioner.* Nov;209:654–60.

———. 1966. "Obesity as a Disease." *Practitioner.* Mar;196:404–9.

———. 1963. "Carbohydrate Addiction." *Practitioner.* Mar;190:358–364.

Lecheminant, J. D., C. A. Gibson, D. K. Sullivan, et al. 2007. "Comparison of a Low Carbohydrate and Low Fat Diet for Weight Maintenance in Overweight or Obese Adults Enrolled in a Clinical Weight Management Program." *Nutrition Journal.* Nov 1;6:36.

National Academy of Sciences, Institute of Medicine, Food and Nutrition Board. 2005. *Dietary Reference Intakes for Energy, Carbohydrate, Fiber, Fat, Fatty Acids, Cholesterol, Protein, and Amino Acids (Macronutrients).* Washington, D.C.: National Academies Press.

Phinney, S. D. "Ketogenic Diets and Physical Performance." *Nutrition & Metabolism.* Aug 17;1(1):2.

Sidbury, J. B., Jr., and R. P. Schwartz. 1975. A Program for Weight Reduction in Children. In *Childhood Obesity,* ed. P. Collip, pp. 65–74: Acton, Mass.: Publishing Sciences Group.

Westman, E. C., W. S. Yancy, J. C. Mavropoulos, M. Marquart, J. R. McDuffie. 2008. "The Effect of a Low-Carbohydrate, Ketogenic Diet versus a Low-Glycemic Index Diet on Glycemic Control in Type 2 Diabetes Mellitus." *Nutrition and Metabolism.* Dec 19;5:36.

Westman, E. C., W. S. Yancy, M. K. Olsen, T. Dudley, J. R. Guyton. 2006. "Effect of a Low-Carbohydrate, Ketogenic Diet Program Compared to a Low-Fat Diet on Fasting Lipoprotein Subclasses." *International Journal of Cardiology.* June 16;110(2):212–16.

Yancy, W. S., M. K. Olsen, J. R. Guyton, R. P. Bakst, E. C. Westman. 2004. "A Low-Carbohydrate, Ketogenic Diet versus a Low-Fat Diet to Treat Obesity

Sources

and Hyperlipidemia: A Randomized, Controlled Trial. *Archives of Internal Medicine.* May 18;140(10):769–77.

Yancy, W. S., M. C. Vernon, and E. C. Westman. 2003. "A Pilot Trial of a Low-Carbohydrate, Ketogenic Diet in Patients with Type 2 Diabetes." *Metabolic Syndrome and Related Disorders.* Sep;1(3):239–43.

Yancy, W. S., E. C. Westman, J. R. McDuffie, et al. 2010. "A Randomized Trial of a Low-Carbohydrate Diet versus Orlistat Plus a Low-Fat Diet for Weight Loss." *Archives of Internal Medicine.* Jan 25;170(2):136–45.

ILLUSTRATION CREDITS

20 "Fat Louisa" photograph. Reprinted from *The Pima Indians*, Frank Russell, page 67. Copyright 1908.

63 Steatopygia photograph. Reprinted from *The Races of Man*, J. Deniker, page 94. Copyright 1900.

64–5 Lean and obese identical twins photographs. Reprinted from *Obesity and Leanness*, Hugo R. Rony, pages 184 and 185. Copyright 1940.

67 Aberdeen Angus photograph. Courtesy of Genus ABS.

67 Jersey cow photograph. By Maggie Murphy, courtesy of Agri-Graphics Ltd.

69 Woman with progressive lipodystrophy photograph. Reprinted from *Obesity and Leanness*, Hugo R. Rony, page 171. Copyright 1940.

70 HIV-related progressive lipodystrophy photographs. Mauss, S. "Lipodystrophy, Metabolic Disorders and Cardiovascular Risk-Complications of Antiretroviral Therapy." *European Pharmacotherapy* 2003, Touch Briefings. © Touch Briefings. Reprinted with permission.

91 The effects of estrogen on LPL illustration. By Ellen Rogers.

98 Author's son, August 2007 and August 2010 photographs. By Larry Lederman.

102 Zucker rat photograph. Courtesy of Charles River Laboratories.

114 Calvin and Hobbes comic strip. Calvin and Hobbes © 1986 Watterson. Reprinted by permission of Universal Uclick. All rights reserved.

117 Fatty acid/tryglyceride illustration. By Ellen Rogers.

122 Effects of insulin on adipose tissue photograph. Courtesy of Informa Healthcare Communications. Reprinted from *Endocrinology: An Integrated Approach*, Stephen Nussey and Saffron Whitehead, page 31. Copyright 2001.

INDEX

Page numbers in *italics* refer to illustrations.
Those followed by *n* indicate a footnote.

Index

Index

cytokines, 197
Czechoslovakia, 29–30

Dancel, Jean-François, 151–2
Davidson, Stanley, 156
Department of Agriculture, U.S.
    (USDA), 44, 57, 136, 160, 165, 181,
    189
desserts, 222
diabetes, 8, 19, 100, 121–2, 132, 150, 152–3,
    177, 182, 195, 197, 198, 200
    and carbohydrate-restricted diets, 203,
      216
    obesity linked to, 41, 84, 135, 196
Diabetes, Coronary Thrombosis and the
    Saccharine Disease (Cleave and
    Campbell), 171
Dictionnaire philosophique (Voltaire),
    16
diet:
    balanced, 173, 174–8
    changes to, 186
    chronic disease associated with,
      168–72
    evolution and, 163–4, 167–8, 176
    healthy, 173–200
    hunter-gatherer, 165–7, 171, 176
    insulin response affected by, 130, 134
    Mediterranean, 25, 189
    official recommendations for, 146,
      160, 162, 165, 167–8, 170
    Western, 167–70
    see also nutrition
Dietary Reference Intakes, 213
diet books, 11, 163, 201–2, 217
Dieter's Dilemma, The (Bennett and
    Gurin), 42
dieting, 33–9, 150
    failure of, 81, 147, 206, 209
diets, carbohydrate-restricted, 201–2
    approaches to, 207–8
    carbohydrate moderation in, 204–10
    clinical trials of, 190–2, 194, 202, 203
    criticisms of, 11–12, 149–50, 153, 160–1,
      162, 172, 173, 174, 175, 178, 217
    doctors' involvement in, 216–17
    effectiveness of, 174, 180, 203, 205
    energy levels and, 209, 211–12
    exercise and, 212, 215
    fat in, 158, 159, 177, 190, 209, 211,
      213–14, 215, 221–2

food labels and, 223, 225
guidelines for, 202, 203, 204–14, 217,
    219–23
and heart disease, 191, 193–4, 203
hunger and, 209, 210, 211, 223
ketosis in, 177–8
menu planner for, 224–5
and metabolic syndrome, 198, 203
non-carbohydrate consumption in,
    210–12
nutrients in, 175–6
pre-1960's recommendation of, 148–9,
    151–9
protein in, 158, 159, 177, 190, 209, 211,
    213–14, 215
reintroduction of carbohydrates in,
    208–9, 210
side effects of, 207, 214–16
testing of, 157–9, 198
for vegetarians, 206–7
diets, high-fat:
    clinical trials of, 190–2, 194, 198
    effects of, 193–4, 198
diets, high-protein, 213
diets, low-calorie:
    carbohydrate restriction in, 175, 188
    clinical trials of, 190
    ineffectiveness of, 140, 147, 158*n*, 174
    weight loss in, 33–8, 140, 144–6, 147,
      158*n*, 174, 188
    weight maintenance following, 38–9
diets, low-fat:
    carbohydrate restriction in, 145, 146
    clinical trials of, 190
    and heart disease, 33, 34*n*, 182, 183–5,
      186, 188
    high protein content in, 213
    promotion of, 180–1, 182, 188, 197
    weight loss in, 144
    women's results in, 33–4
digestion, 114–15, 123, 125, 135, 136, 141
    see also metabolism
disease, chronic, 8, 164, 184
    modern diet associated with, 168–72
    obesity linked to, 5, 41, 49, 84, 135,
      179, 182, 195, 196, 197, 198, 199, 200
    see also metabolic syndrome; *specific*
      diseases
Dobyns, Henry, 23
Donaldson, Blake, 163, 164, 179, 216*n*
Dr. Atkins' Diet Revolution, 190, 201

Index

drugs:
anti-retroviral, 70
appetite-suppressing, 38
and carbohydrate-restricted diets, 216,
223
cholesterol-lowering, 182–3, 186
Du Bois, Eugene, 59–60
Duke University Medical Center, 202,
219
DuPont Company, 157, 158, 163*n*

Eades, Michael and Mary Dan, 204
eating:
insulin secretion in response to,
114–15, 123, 141
in moderation, 4, 6, 60–1, 84, 104–5,
128, 211
see also appetite; diet; overeating
Eco, Umberto, 53
eggs, 219
electrolyte imbalances, 215
endocrinology, 107, 108, 112, 159
Endocrinology: An Integrated Approach
(Nussly and Whitehead), 121
energy:
body fat requirements of, 103–4, 126
calorie intake as dependent on, 77–9,
90, 92, 101, 104, 128, 209
on carbohydrate-restricted diets, 209,
211–12
in cells, 78, 79, 94, 114, 115, 118, 126,
128, 131, 140, 214
conservation of, 73–4, 97–8
fat cells' storage of, 113–14, 115–16, 118,
123–4, 126
nutrient requirements for, 147
use of, 141
see also calories; exercise; inactivity;
nutrients
enzymes, 127, 132, 137
fat tissue regulated by, 10, 92, 93, 105,
109, 118–21, 127, 204
epilepsy, 178
Ernst, Nancy, 181
estrogen, 90–2, 91, 94, 119, 204
Europe, pre-WWII obesity paradigm in,
9, 62–3, 106–8, 149–59
evolution, 96, 163–4, 167–8, 176
exercise, 40–56
assumptions about, 46–7, 52–4, 55

on carbohydrate-restricted diets, 212,
215
changing view of, 49–54
historical views on, 47–8
hunger caused by, 40, 47, 48, 50, 53,
78, 120, 212
ineffectiveness of, 6–7, 44–5, 47–8, 52,
54–6, 119–20, 147
metabolic effect of, 119–20
metabolism supporting, 104–5
official guidelines on, 7, 43–4, 51, 55
scientific studies of, 44–5, 52, 53–4,
55–6
and weight loss, 52, 146–7, 212
and weight maintenance, 44–6
see also "calories-in/calories-out"
paradigm; inactivity; physical
labor

fasting, 158*n*, 205
fat, body:
abdominal, 33, 62, 119, 120, 195, 197
burning of, 91, 115–16, 119, 120, 121,
124, 125–6, 174, 177, 207, 208, 211,
212, 214
calories in, 34, 58
distribution of, 62–3, 68–71, 94, 119
energy required for, 103–4, 126
formation of, 152, 197
genetic influence on, 63, 63, 64, 67,
94, 107, 109, 127, 132
storage of, 113–17, 117, 118, 119, 120,
123, 124, 125–6, 128*n*, 129, 130, 138
see also fatty acids; obesity;
triglycerides; weight loss
fat, dietary, 144, 152, 174
calories in, 180
in carbohydrate-restricted diets, 158,
159, 177, 190, 209, 211, 213–14, 215,
221–2
essential, 176
HDL cholesterol raised by, 188, 189,
190, 192, 194, 198
heart disease allegedly linked to, 24,
160–2, 172, 173, 178–86
in hunter-gatherer diets, 165–6
ketone synthesis from, 177
metabolism of, 114, 115, 118, 123, 142,
206
nutrients in, 180

Index

official recommendations for, 146n,
160, 162, 165, 180–1, 182, 185, 188
restriction of, 146, 147, 179
saturated, 161, 175, 178, 179, 180, 181,
182–6, 188, 189, 190, 192, 195, 196,
213
triglyceride level unaffected by, 187
types of, 189
see also diets, low-fat
fat cells:
cholesterol stored in, 215n
creation of, 121
fat accumulation in, 91–2, 97, 114,
115–16, 117, 117, 118, 119, 120, 121, 123,
124, 128n, 129, 130, 131, 134, 137, 138,
142, 147, 197
fat release from, 120, 121, 123, 124, 125,
126, 177
fuel provided by, 113–14, 115–16, 118,
123–4, 126, 211
insulin resistance in, 129, 130, 131
triglyceride breakdown in, 120–1, 124
triglyceride construction in, 117, 117,
121, 123
fat metabolism, 113–18
fat regulation, 9–10, 89–105, 112–26
in animals, 95–6, 99–104
diet as influencing, 112, 147, 206
genetic component of, 63, 63, 64, 67,
94, 107, 109, 127, 132, 204
hormones' involvement in, 9–10, 92,
93, 101, 105, 109, 114–15, 118–26,
127–30, 204
pre-1960s views on, 106–11
fatty acids, 139, 177
burning of, 116, 120, 123, 124, 176
release of, 118, 120, 121, 123, 124, 126,
215n
storage of, 116, 117, 117, 119, 120, 121,
123, 141
fatty liver disease, 138, 139, 200
fiber, 135, 145, 166, 221, 225
fish, 165, 219
Flier, Jeffrey, 37, 78, 79, 81
flour, refined, 134
*Food, Nutrition, Physical Activity and
the Prevention of Cancer*, 199
Food Guide Pyramid, 160, 165
Foucault's Pendulum (Eco), 53
French, James, 154

fructose, 114, 123n, 136–8, 142, 145
see also high-fructose corn syrup
fruit, 136, 137, 166–7, 170, 176

Gardiner-Hill, H., 154
Gardner, Christopher, 192, 194
Gehrmann, George, 157
genes, 94, 102, 132, 187
body type determined by, 63, 64, 67
diet and, 164, 167–8
early study of, 107, 108
fat regulation influenced by, 107, 109,
127, 204
Gladwell, Malcolm, 8
glucose, 117, 132, 139, 177
insulin secreted in response to, 115,
123, 129, 134, 142
metabolism of, 114, 115, 121, 123, 129,
130, 134, 137, 138, 141, 142, 176, 214
glucose intolerance, 131, 195
glycemic index, 135n, 166, 206
glycerol, 116, 117, 121, 177
glycogen, 115, 118, 128n, 130, 142
gout, 197, 200
Grafe, Erich, 68
Greene, Raymond, 155, 203
Griffin, John, 21
growth, 9, 93, 98–9, 105
growth factor, 10, 199
Gurin, Joel, 42

Handbook of Obesity (Bray, Bouchard,
and James), 37, 54
Handbook of Physiology, 161
Hanssen, Per, 157, 174
Harvey, William, 152–3
heart disease, 62, 96
carbohydrate-restricted diets and, 191,
193–4, 203
and carbohydrates, 180, 200
cholesterol-lowering drugs and, 183,
186
HDL cholesterol and, 187–90, 193–4
increased incidence of, 181, 182
low-fat diets and, 33, 34n, 182, 183–5,
186, 188
obesity linked to, 41, 179, 182, 196
risk factors for, 187–90, 191, 193–4,
195, 196–7; *see also* metabolic
syndrome

Index

Index

mayonnaise, 221
meat, 160, 165, 166, 170–1, 175–6
  on carbohydrate-restricted diet, 219, 225
  unlimited consumption of, 152, 154, 163, 192, 202
medical establishment:
  dietary fat condemned by, 180
  heart disease advice from, 178–9, 180–1, 185, 188
  obesity advice from, 5, 6, 8, 37–8, 75, 76, 79, 82–3, 84, 92–3, 112, 136, 149–50, 153, 159–62, 197–8, 216
  pre-WWII obesity research ignored by, 108
  see also nutrition; public health
men, fat distribution in, 68, 94, 119
menopause, 119
Metabolic Diseases and Their Treatment (Grafe), 68
metabolic syndrome, 195–200, 203
metabolism, 79, 108, 131, 195
  of carbohydrates, 114, 115, 123, 124, 126, 128–9, 130, 134–9
Mueller, William, 28
muscle, 54, 105, 126
  loss of, 34, 74n, 103, 212
muscle cells:
  fat burning in, 91, 119, 120, 128, 130
  glycogen stored in, 115, 128, 130
  insulin resistance in, 129, 130, 131, 138, 195
  protein in, 118, 120, 126, 142, 147

National Heart, Lung, and Blood Institute (NHLBI), 180–1, 182–3
National Institutes of Health, 20, 33, 52, 59, 75, 76, 196
Native Americans, 171
  obesity among, 19–24, 25–6, 27, 28
Nestle, Marion, 17
Newburgh, Louis, 48, 82, 107, 108
Noorden, Carl von, 55, 72
North Carolina, 27
nutrients, 147, 175, 180
nutrition, 108, 150, 165
  modern recommendations for, 49, 113–14, 136, 150, 170, 172, 175, 176–7, 178, 188
  scientific evidence in, 16, 51, 172

transition in, 168, 171–2
see also diet

obesity:
  in animals, 89–90, 95, 100–3
  assumptions about, 29, 49, 75–6
  behavioral view of, 80–6, 93, 108, 110–11, 159
  cancer associated with, 41, 199, 200
  causes of, 10, 76, 90, 93, 94, 96–7, 125, 126, 128, 144, 200, 201
  changing view of, 159–62
  in children, 18, 24, 25–6, 131–3, 210
  chronic disease linked to, 5, 41, 49, 84, 135, 179, 182, 195, 196, 197, 198, 199, 200
  consequences of, 4, 35, 80, 110–11
  in Depression era, 3–4, 19
  diabetes linked to, 41, 84, 135, 195, 196
  as form of malnutrition, 29–30
  heart disease linked to, 41, 179, 182, 196
  malnutrition coexisting with, 24–8, 30, 31, 61, 104, 113–14
  medical advice about, 5, 6, 8, 37–8, 75, 76, 79, 82–3, 84, 92–3, 112, 136, 149–50, 153, 159–62, 197–8, 216
  among Native Americans, 19–24, 20
  poverty linked to, 18–29, 30, 31, 41–2, 104, 135
  pre-1960s views on, 9, 62–3, 106–8, 149–59, 203
  predisposition to, 63, 83, 94, 97, 127–33, 134, 140, 142, 143
  science of, 11–12, 16–17, 73, 81, 112–25, 159, 161, 195, 203, 217
  see also "calories-in/calories-out" paradigm; fat, body; weight loss
Obesity, or Excessive Corpulence (Dancel), 151
obesity epidemic, 7–8, 17–20, 42–3, 132, 133, 150, 182
Ohlson, Margaret, 157, 158
oleic acid, 189
olives, olive oil, 189, 221
Ornish, Dean, 144, 145, 150
Ornish diet, 191
Osler, William, 154
ovaries, 89, 90, 92

Index

overeating:
assumptions about, 17, 81, 82, 197
causes of, 9, 90, 92, 97–9, 101, 103,
105, 111, 126
by children, 4, 9
see also "calories-in/calories-out"
paradigm
oxidative stress, 197

pancreas, 114, 129, 132, 195
Passmore, Reginald, 156
Pavlov, Ivan, 141
Pennington, Alfred, 157, 158, 163n
Phinney, Stephen, 203, 204, 210, 216
physical labor:
obesity coincident with, 22, 27, 29,
41–2
see also exercise
physiology, 109, 159
Physiology of Taste, The (Brillat-
Savarin), 148
pickles, 221
Pima, 19–23, 20, 25–6, 169
Pi-Sunyer, Xavier, 52
Pollan, Michael, 5, 25, 34, 168, 171
poultry, 219
poverty:
carbohydrate-rich diets and, 135, 138
obesity linked to, 18–29, 30, 31, 41–2,
104, 135
Practice of Endocrinology, The (Greene
et al.), 155, 203
Practice of Medicine, The (Tanner), 151
pregnancy, 119, 132
Principles and Practice of Medicine, The
(Osler), 154
progressive lipodystrophy, 68–70, 69
"Proposals for Nutritional Guidelines
for Health Education in Britain,"
162
protein:
body fat not caused by, 144, 147, 152
in muscle cells, 118, 120, 126, 142
storage of, 118, 126, 142
protein, dietary, 118, 142, 147, 166, 169,
174, 179, 180
in carbohydrate-restricted diets, 158,
159, 177, 190, 209, 211, 213–14, 215
official recommendations for, 146n,
165, 213
see also meat

Protein Power (Eades and Eades), 201,
204
puberty, 68, 99
public health, 31, 164
modern recommendations in, 136,
159, 170, 188, 199–200
scientific evidence in, 16, 185, 217

Ranson, Stephen, 101
rats, obesity in, 89–90, 102–3
Reaven, Gerald, 196, 198
Renold, Albert, 116
Richards, Rolf, 28, 30, 135
Rifkind, Basil, 183
Rony, Hugo, 48, 108n, 110n
Rose, Geoffrey, 164, 165
Rosedale, Ron, 202
running, 42–3, 45–6, 52
Russell, Frank, 20, 20, 22

science, 16
of heart disease, 185–6, 193–4
of obesity, 11–12, 16–17, 73, 81, 112–25,
159, 161, 195, 203, 217
"Sick Individuals and Sick Populations"
(Rose), 164
Sidbury, James, Jr., 210
Sioux, 23–4, 30
sleep, 115, 125, 177
snacks, 212, 221
sodium, 197, 215–16
soft drinks, 136, 137, 145
Sontag, Susan, 85
soy sauce, 221
Spock, Benjamin, 156
Stanford University A to Z Trial, 144,
191–2, 194
starches, 134, 137, 145, 152
avoidance of, 202, 221, 225
see also carbohydrate-rich foods
starvation, in Zucker rats, 102–3
steatopygia, 62, 63, 94
Stern, Judith, 53
"Strategy of Prevention" (Rose), 164
stress, 124
stroke, 184, 195
Stunkard, Albert, 35, 36
sucrose, 136–7, 196
sugars, 136–8, 152, 196
addiction to, 142–3, 209–10
avoidance of, 202, 204, 221, 225

Index

A Note About the Author

Gary Taubes is the author of *Good Calories, Bad Calories: Challenging the Conventional Wisdom on Diet, Weight Control, and Disease*. He is a contributing correspondent for *Science* magazine, and a Robert Wood Johnson Foundation investigator in health policy research at the University of California, Berkeley, School of Public Health. His articles about science, medicine, and health have appeared in *Discover*, *The Atlantic*, and *The New York Times Magazine*, among other publications. He has won three Science-in-Society Journalism Awards, given by the National Association of Science Writers—the only print journalist so recognized—as well as awards from the Pan American Health Organization, the American Institute of Physics, and the American Physical Society. His writing was selected for *The Best American Science Writing 2002*, *The Best of the Best of American Science Writing*, and *The Best American Science and Nature Writing 2000 and 2003*. He is also the author of *Bad Science* and *Nobel Dreams*. He was educated at Harvard, Stanford, and Columbia. He lives in Berkeley, California, with his wife and two sons.

A Note on the Type

The text of this book was set in Electra, a typeface designed by W. A. Dwiggins (1880–1956). This face cannot be classified as either modern or old style. It is not based on any historical model, nor does it echo any particular period or style. It avoids the extreme contrasts between thick and thin elements that mark most modern faces, and it attempts to give a feeling of fluidity, power, and speed.

Composed by North Market Street Graphics,
Lancaster, Pennsylvania
Printed and bound by RR Donnelley,
Harrisonburg, Virginia
Designed by Virginia Tan